Cont

'O, *full of scorpions is my mind…*'

William Shakespeare, *Macbeth*

'Who knows
The hot stung days
And brittle cold nights
Of keeping a great poison pure.'

J. Michael Yates, extract from 'Scorpion'

AUTHOR'S NOTE

Before we begin, I want to inform you that this book contains descriptions of compulsive rituals and obsessive thought cycles, which are intended to provide an immersive experience of OCD, but which those with the condition could find distressing or disruptive to their own recovery, should they be vulnerable to adopting the compulsions of others. Please take care when reading.

Prologue

My mind is full of scorpions. Devious, nimble little beasts that have occupied my head for the best part of thirty years. A cerebral itch, impossible to scratch. They wield their own special power over my brain, shaping the architecture and rhythm of my thoughts. An immovable nest, weighing heavy in my skull.

Small armoured bodies scuttle along an intricate web of neural pathways, disturbing the delicate flow of logical thought. Tempered chaos in perpetual motion.

I know these creatures well, but they know me better. There is a ferocious edge to their loyalty, yet something hollow lurks in their promise to keep me safe. I am their dutiful puppet, stuck inside an endless loop of sleepless nights and watchful days. I carry my secret quietly, afraid to expose these wayward sentries. The gatekeepers of my sanity.

They answer to another name, this nest of scorpions, the writhing black mass that lives inside my head:

Obsessive-
                    Compulsive
            Disorder.

Imagine a day, much like today, where you find yourself inside a room. Not unlike the room you inhabit as you read these words. Perhaps you are cooking, or working, or sitting with friends. You become aware of something stealing into your peripheral vision, disrupting an otherwise harmonious scene. Something you are scared of. For argument's sake, let's say it's a large, albeit harmless, spider. It has entered your sphere and now begins to navigate the room with a volatile unpredictability. You can try to ignore it as you go about your business, maybe you even succeed for a while, but you are always *aware* that it is there. You watch its every move, and it watches yours. Now, why not add an element of danger? It is not a spider that has wandered into your domain, but a scorpion. Bigger and tougher and faster than a spider, its curved tail is armed with a deadly sting. You cannot fail to ignore the presence of this unwelcome visitor. As you talk with your friends, it is in the room. As you prepare your dinner, it is in the room. As you scan these lines, *it is in the room.* Lose sight of it and a panic begins to take hold. Never let your eyes leave its glistening form and your life stands frozen in time. To live a contented life alongside an uncaged scorpion requires a delicate balance of trust, will and surrender. This is the image I return to when attempting to articulate my experience of living with obsessive compulsive disorder (OCD).

OCD is a mental illness that affects around 2 per cent of the global population, but the proportion of people touched by it is far higher. A condition that causes obsessive, unwanted thoughts and repetitive behaviours known as compulsions, it is often described as a 'silent' illness, carrying with it a lot of shame, stigma and misconception. It is common, and relatively easy, for sufferers to disguise or hide it due to the internal nature of the intrusive thoughts and the embarrassment brought about by irrational or unusual compulsions.

As a society, we often inadvertently classify certain mental health disorders as less acute than others, in particular OCD. It is sadly still trivialised by the media and many people falsely believe that it can be filed under a personality type characterised by traits or quirks such as liking things to be clean or being concerned with order. There is a plethora of novelty merchandise available to buy, branding their owner as 'a little bit OCD'. I have a coffee mug that I received as a Christmas present many years ago in my own kitchen cupboard that has the words OBSESSIVE COMPULSIVE emblazoned across it in bright pink letters. It is hard to imagine a line of gift items with ANOREXIA or PTSD boldly stamped upon them for all to see. So why is OCD continually used as a shorthand for light-hearted craziness, or categorised as one of the more comic disorders of the mind?

The truth is that this condition can devastate people's lives, leading to job loss, relationship breakdown and total isolation, as well as, in more severe cases, suicide. Diagnosis is often reached much later than it should be for numerous reasons, be that social, cultural or familial, but from my own experience I know that it was a condition that my family and I had heard very little about when I was growing up, let alone felt able to seek help for. Thankfully, the conversation around mental health has opened up a lot since I was a child, but to me it feels as though OCD is still relatively misunderstood and needs to be explored further, allowing it the same opportunity for research and treatment as other more widely discussed mental health conditions such as anxiety or depression.

When I first began to navigate what it meant to have obsessive compulsive disorder, I longed for someone to guide me through the knot of disjointed thinking. A beacon of hope to look up to, who could demonstrate how I might find my way amongst the scorpions that were inhabiting my brain. I hope that by talking honestly and specifically about the problems I have faced living with OCD, I can help someone, in some small way, not to feel so helpless or alone.

For as long as I can remember I have struggled with obsessive thoughts, checking compulsions, and an extreme fear of vomiting. Manifesting and evolving in different ways at each stage of my life, OCD has affected me with varying levels of severity over the years. Something rarely talked about with anyone other than family or friends, I recently made the decision to discuss my experience publicly and was overwhelmed by the response I received. I realised how many people are still too afraid to talk about it, and as a result are not receiving the help that they desperately need. When I was an oblivious pre-teen discovering the intricacies of a disorder I knew nothing about, I longed to hear stories about people who thought the way that I did. The few legends available to me always seemed so sensationalised and extreme in nature. The cripplingly restrictive lifestyle of eccentric businessman and film tycoon Howard Hughes was a well-worn example of a what it meant to have OCD. Some of his rumoured behaviours, such as keeping bottles of his own urine and wearing tissue boxes on his feet to avoid contamination, seemed to push me so far from any sense of understanding that I was too terrified to even try to relate.

It took time for me to discover my own icon, found by chance aged twenty-two, when gazing upon images of the world's most famous tomb – that belonging to Tutankhamun. In Egyptian mythology there is a goddess called Serket. She is one of the four goddesses who adorns the canopic shrine of the boy pharaoh, and is most commonly depicted as a woman with a scorpion crowning her head. She serves to watch over and heal those suffering from a deadly sting. Not only a scorpion wielder, but a protector too, able to mitigate this mighty force, both sinister and benignant. This goddess with her scorpion crown compelled me to one day share my own scorpions with the world, a steadfast reminder of the loads we carry with us. Exposing and empowering. Mundane and absurd.

The stories we tell ourselves and others about obsessive compulsive disorder are beginning to change. They are more honest, more nuanced, and whilst the routines may feel familiar, each story remains unique. To those who recognise themselves in some of the rituals or thought patterns in this book, I hope that it will mean as much to you as it would have meant to me all those years ago, and I can assure you that it is possible to lead a happy, functioning existence as an obsessive-compulsive person.

Chapter One

GESTATION

'These hardy, adaptable arthropods have been
around for hundreds of millions of years, and
they are nothing if not survivors.'

National Geographic

I have always hated going to bed. Like most eleven-year-olds, I'd attempt to use all manner of different distractions to impede this nightly fate as dusk began its languid approach. One particularly wet Sunday evening, I had exhausted all my usual sleep-avoidance tactics: making myself small and uninteresting so as not to be noticed, striking up impossibly long conversations in which all my replies ended with questions. My younger brother was already in bed after having endured a day of makeovers at the behest of his sisters, so only the two of us remained downstairs, as still and quiet as church mice. Being the middle child, I was given the marching orders first by my father, at a frankly tyrannical 8.30pm. He pretended not to see the expression I affixed to my face (in acknowledge-ment of the injustice): screwing up my nose and forcing my eyes into a gloomy squint. I get my dark eyes from him, but not my height. A true perfectionist, who winces at swearwords, he is generous, fiercely loyal, and every-one's idea of a dream neighbour. Unfazed by the big things, fazed by the small, he is always last to bed at a party. On this occasion, I decided against arguing my case and instead wished the room a sulky goodnight. I caught my sister's eye and she offered a sympathetic smile, like a gymnast witnessing a teammate stumble on the final pose. We were even dressed alike, in thick fluffy dressing gowns and padded socks, despite our house always being several degrees too warm, a fact that my parents will claim until their dying day is due to some defect with the radiators, rather than a penchant for the subtropical.

I crawled up the stairs to my room on all-fours to prolong the journey, and stopped just short of my bedroom door, a jaded sigh escaping me as I placed my hand on the doorknob. I peered inside, resisting the urge to flick on the light switch, an act that I'd spent months convincing myself must not only be delayed each night, but more importantly, earned. I braced myself for the task ahead, knowing it would require my undivided attention – a small house accommodating five human beings (three under thirteen) was not the ideal space in which to find long stretches of undisturbed peace and quiet. Peace and quiet was all I needed. And time, because as always, what I had to do was going to take a lot of it.

Around half an hour later, I heard a pair of weary legs ascend the steps towards the landing. My mother startled, surprised to find me still awake and standing motionless at the threshold of my room with the door barely ajar, focusing intently on something inside. She is a tall, fair-haired woman who carries the seaside in her blood and has always looked younger than her years. A part-time confidante and full-time worrier, she puts family above everything and begins half of all sentences with 'sorry'.

'What are you doing?' she said, a hint of alarm in her voice. 'Haven't you gone to bed yet?'

'I'm doing my routine,' I answered abruptly, acutely aware that the interruption meant I would have to start all over again. She looked at me in confusion.

'What routine?'

The winter prior to this, I had contracted a particularly nasty stomach bug that had annihilated me for four long, miserable days. The virus had spread like wildfire through my Year 6 class, forcing me to set up camp in the room nearest the bathroom at my grandparents' house. For reasons that escape me now, they shared the caretaking with my mother, and as a result, half of my week was spent lounging feebly across their florid sofa attempting to distract myself with cartoon skeletons and my grandad's gleefully delivered jokes – courtesy of *Reader's Digest*. Meanwhile, I was force-fed a smorgasbord of mint humbugs, shredded marmalade and anaemic tinned carrots, alongside the flat Coca-Cola prescribed by my well-meaning grand-mother, which all came shooting through my nose into the kitchen sink at regular intervals when I failed to make it to the toilet in time.

I soon recovered, however, as almost all children do, quickly and entirely, and went about my business, revelling in the unbridled chaos of Christmas. The overwhelming but short-lived horror that spans the duration of any childhood winter vomiting bug was soon forgotten and the second term of my final year at primary started as uneventfully as all the others had.

The ordeal that followed began on a car journey to school one spring morning.

We were sat in a traffic jam snaking the length of a country road that bridged the long and verdant gap between two West Country villages. My mother, with endless reserves of patience, was refereeing a territorial spat between my brother and sister in the back regarding thighs crossing car-seat boundary lines, whilst I kept myself busy up front cultivating the requisite amount of dread to confess my current physical state.

'I feel sick,' I mumbled cautiously. (There is nothing like announcing nausea to accelerate the feeling tenfold.) Mum flicked the radio off and put her hand to my forehead. I could feel a faint air of panic from my siblings behind me.

'You do look a bit peaky. Maybe it's travel sickness?' she offered hopefully. 'I'll wind the window down.'

'No, it's not that. It can't be, I'm in the front.' Mum nodded at this, a firm believer in the recognised prevention and age-old cure of 'sitting in the front' for the affliction that plagued two of her three children. That unrelenting queasiness caused by serpentine country lanes or the back seats of cramped leathery cars.

'Shall I pull over?' she suggested, looking at me like I was an unexploded bomb.

I nodded defeatedly, awash with injustice that I'd managed to catch yet another virus so soon after my recent decimation, and she pulled the car onto the grassy ridge bordering the road. In full view of the building traffic, I felt a steady stream of nosy, sympathetic eyes fall on me as I opened the door and leaned weakly out from the side of the car.

'Are you alright?' Mum asked after several dedicated minutes of back-rubbing and comforting tuts. 'Do you think you're going to be sick or should I keep on driving?'

As utterly pathetic as I felt, my stomach had developed a severe case of stage fright and nothing actually appeared to be happening. The clock on the dashboard of our green Renault (still set to British Summer Time from the previous year) was ticking at what felt like double speed, and, as I hated being late as much as I hated going to bed, I finally agreed to let my mother drive on towards school, goaded by the impending threat of more cars and mocking faces.

For the remainder of our seemingly endless journey, my siblings were treated to a slew of pitiful declarations – a running commentary of my nausea. Window down, window up, window down, window up. Everyone in the vehicle was engaged in the frantic search for a suitable vessel into which I could vomit, should the moment eventually strike.

We arrived outside the school gates before anyone managed to locate such a vessel, and my sister and brother made a swift exit, hellbent on avoiding the looming possibility of hot-boxing our family car with a potent mix of stomach acid and hysteria. I, however, stayed rooted to the spot and waited until they were well out of sight before casting a forlorn look to my mother in the driver's seat.

'I don't want to go in, I still feel sick.' We heard the school bell ring out and watched two lines begin to form in the playground – one for the boys, another for the girls – as a teacher with thinning hair and small round glasses stood poised, a whistle between his lips.

'OK, darling, I'll take you home. You don't look very well,' she concluded, and we began the endless drive home in anticipatory silence. Windows down.

The days afterwards played out much the same as this first sombre journey. Nausea became a distressingly predictable part of my day, rushing over me in waves from the moment I woke up until the moment I dragged myself back to bed again. This unresolved nausea was a constant needling presence, persistent yet vomit-less. Each morning of the school run, whether I was commandeering the front seat or sandwiched between my siblings on the familiar route through the countryside, ended in exactly the same way. The inevitable queasiness eventually gave way to tears at the school gate, pleading not to go in. A clear absence of any visible symptoms left me powerless to substantiate my condition as the days rolled over into a second week, and as two weeks became three and the exhaustion became undeniable to myself and my parents, I was taken to the local doctor's surgery to see our family GP.

'So she's never actually sick?' enquired Dr G, choosing to direct this to the room rather than the little girl sat before him, as he jotted another illegible squiggle onto his notepad. I pitched him at double the age he actually was, on account of the grey beginning to tinge the roots of his hair, and possessing the type of wise, caramel voice bestowed upon healthcare professionals of a longstanding stature.

My mother had interlaced her fingers to stop them from fidgeting as my eyes found the miniature cardboard tray lying in my lap, designed to catch small trickles of vomit from only the most delicate of regurgitators. I grimaced as I found myself wondering exactly how many pools of vomit had been cleaned from the floor of this room.

'No, she just *feels* sick, all the time. She hardly eats and spends all day in bed. Look how much weight she's lost!'

'Hmmm.' Dr G chewed his lip, clicking through several web pages on his new computer, which took up half the space on his desk. A handful of gargantuan desktops had recently appeared at our local general practice, and I got the distinct impression that he would rather be playing solitaire than puzzling over my indeterminate repertoire of symptoms. His eyes didn't leave the screen as he suggested, 'Perhaps there's something going on at school? Something Tuppence is ... worried about?'

'Well, she's not being bullied or anything, if that's what you mean,' Mum usurped, turning to me for confirmation. 'Are you? You must tell me if you are —'

'No,' I cut her off quickly. 'I love school. I want to go back.'

I was telling the truth, despite the hand-scrawled letter containing a smeared bogey that had been passed to me by a smirking Sally P in biology a few weeks earlier, or the scar on my hand from when she'd pushed me into a white-hot Bunsen burner. It was easy to reframe these events as a series of 'friendship tests' that each of the three girls in our group had to pass in order to prove their allegiance to the others. Although it did seem odd that I was the only one being tested and that Sally was the only one setting these tests, but as I often did when faced with other people's logic, I decided to trust blindly in her methods. At a weekend sleepover she'd once ordered me to drink a cocktail made from milk, orange juice and Pepsi, before proceeding to do so herself and promptly vomiting into the kitchen sink. (It was the zip-line that Sally constructed from her bedroom window to the garden shed whilst her parents were out – touted as the only way in which I was allowed to leave her house that evening – that finally made me hesitate and question these absurd demonstrations of loyalty.)

Despite those minor occurrences, I realised, sitting quietly in the doctor's office, that I worried constantly about these friends who hadn't noticed I was gone, about what I was missing, and how far I was falling behind with my work. My mother too was exhausted with worry and pressed Dr G to investigate further.

We were referred to a specialist at our local children's hospital, who took us through a variety of possible options, ranging from glandular fever to 'attention-seeking', none of which could be supported by enough clinical or observational evidence to make a credible diagnosis. There were blood tests, heart checks, physical examinations, questionnaires, further investigations into balance/fitness/co-ordination/diet/social habits. All the while I was trying my hardest to overcome the sickness, and continued to venture reluctantly into the classroom each day, often to be sent home again by lunchtime. Time behind my desk became a distant memory, whilst my visits to the school nurse became reliably frequent, and before long she could tell the time almost to the minute by the sound of my gentle knocking on her door, my safe haven at thirty-five minutes past eleven, when the bell rang out for our first break of the day. Once inside, I'd beg for her to call home and ask someone to collect me. I lay in my designated place on her small fold-up bed and listened to the muffled sound of my mother's voice on the other end of the line, deciding my fate for the day from some far-off realm: that mysterious childless place that parents disappear to between the hours of eight o'clock and three o'clock. I reassured myself that, although I was losing hours of learning to my new pastime of keeping the school nurse company, I had studied the St John Ambulance poster on the wall opposite my sickbed in such extensive detail that I was convinced that if all else failed and I couldn't return to full time education, I could at least get work as a junior paramedic. Eventually the nurse stopped calling home, because I stopped coming to school. The complexities of structuring your day around a poorly child turned into an organisational feat too great for my parents to predict, and soon it was decided that I should stay at home until we could work out exactly what was wrong with me. After more tests and multiple lengthy discussions – and in the absence of any clear parameters – I was diagnosed by the hospital with myalgic encephalomyelitis (ME) or chronic fatigue syndrome, as it is also known. ME/CFS is one of those mysterious conditions often landed upon as a last-resort diagnosis, by way of ruling out every other possible illness in the world. Described somewhat unhelpfully by the NHS as 'a long-term condition with a wide range of symptoms', the lack of research into this illness is notable, and undermines the sheer intensity of said 'wide range of symptoms'. Treatment options, we soon learned, were frustratingly vague.

Shortly after we received this news, I was back at home listening from my hiding place at the top of the stairs as my parents conferred in the hallway. My mother had just come off the phone to a senior consultant at the Bristol Children's Hospital, and I could hear that she'd been crying.

'He said she might not get better – it can last for years apparently,' she relayed between sobs. 'Sometimes even a lifetime! They don't really know how to treat it, so we just have to wait, and *hope* she recovers. She doesn't want to go out and play or do anything, he said she might not even be able to carry her own bags or go back to school or—'

I lost the remainder of my prognosis to whispers and tears. I tuned back in to the conversation in time for my father's attempt to counter her distress with a steady flow of logic. A curious feeling of indifference washed over me as I made my way back to bed for another cycle of unrefreshing sleep, and I was surprised to acknowledge that, regardless of the potential seriousness of my condition, I didn't have an ounce of energy left to care.

So began a convalescence worthy of the sickly younger sister in a Victorian Gothic novel, as I observed my gradual decline from the outside. My diagnosis came shortly before Easter, and instead of unleashing my insatiable sweet tooth onto the chocolate egg population of Somerset, I watched my body shrink rapidly to half its usual size, and as the weeks continued on, a thick fog began to settle around my brain.

Eating became virtually impossible and I survived on minuscule portions of dry toast, Rich Tea biscuits and lemonade. We are a family of big eaters. Food-worshippers. It was the only time in my life I have ever lost my appetite and it drained every last drop of energy from my body. With little physical drive and no mealtimes to punctuate the ennui of my days I became an empty shell, a poor imitation of my former spritely self. The few mornings that I had managed to make it into the car and attempt the arduous journey into school, I moved in agonising slow motion. The action of slipping a school shirt gently around my skeletal shoulders made my arms feel like lead as I struggled to catch shallow breaths. Roving around the house – no matter how small the distance – was like wading through sticky mud, and as the days slipped by in a repetitive blur, I found no better solution than to confine myself to my room and stare.

For the next four achingly slow months I embarked unwittingly on a life lived solely inside my head. With nothing but books, films, bed and boredom for company, I retreated to a dreamlike interior world. Sleepwalking through the monotonous days, I was afraid to leave the house – imagining a hostile universe outside my front door, full of danger and possibility. The range of activities available to me inside of those four walls, however, were decidedly limited. I became obsessed with doo-wop music, and spent the hours I was awake watching old Hollywood films with my mother, who noted any improvement – however minimal – with a hope bordering on despair. My friends no longer asked if I was coming out to play, and the remaining pockets of confidence I had worked so hard to cultivate slowly faded to nothing.

As my illness continued into its fifth month, the end of the summer fast approaching, I had learned how to best conserve my energy when faced with overwhelming fatigue, and how to create my own adventures within the constructs of an isolated mind. With time passing at the characteristically sedate pace of childhood, I wondered if this state of being might become the dependable bedrock of my existence. I would become an exhausted adult, as seamlessly as I had become an exhausted child. But just as I had come to accept this new, fragile way of life, something began to change. With no conceivable inter-vention – medical or otherwise – and in the subtlest of ways, measured in fractions of a millimetre, I started to feel better. My parents watched, quietly hopeful, as each day I woke up a little bit brighter, a little more connected to the world around me. Days soon became weeks and as I started to sleep less, my mother could sleep more, allowing herself the long-awaited luxury of a night free from restless anxiety. The blood seemed to pump through my veins with a renewed purpose, the heaviness gradually lifted from my bones so I could walk further, stay awake longer, and feel like a child again. The last week of the school holidays was drawing nearer and it became a very real possibility that I might finally return to education for the start of my first secondary school term. My parents' joy and disbelief was matched only by mine, when slowly but surely, my appetite returned. The relief I felt was all-encompassing when my nausea began to subside, and almost without realising, the days fell away behind me and I found that I was stronger, happier and *hungrier*. Not only for food, but for an entirely new kind of existence. I wanted to move and play and discover myself anew. Finding the courage to embrace real life after such a long hiatus was the hardest part of my re-emerging into the world. And re-emerge I did, careful but determined, like a butterfly bursting from its pupa, fluttering nervously into an exhilarating new sphere. One in which I could take back control of my shattered body and delicate mind.

...Then the scorpions arrived.

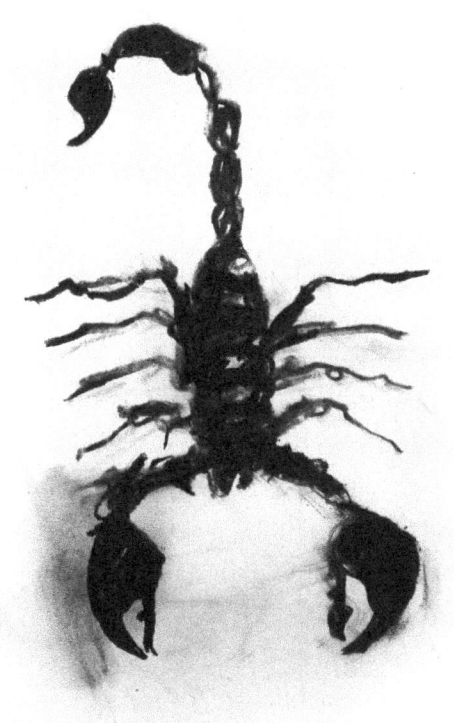

I didn't notice them at first, taking root in the smallest, darkest corner of my mind. Whilst I was losing myself to months of perpetual slumber, a change was taking place inside my head. A birth.

They grew quietly. Secretly. Flourishing and multiplying as I unknowingly provided them with the optimal conditions in which to evolve. A safe and delicate space to call home in the shadows of my cranial womb, their careful development undisturbed by the discord of a busy life. Devoid of thoughts nurtured by a stimulated mind, I offered these creatures the open reins to a pliable young brain. They worked tirelessly to construct their intricate nest, mapping the complex system of neural pathways twisting and intersecting in the soft tissue beneath my skull. And all the time, I was watching. The smallest actions and subtlest of thoughts became gigantic in my minuscule world. Nothing was important, yet everything was loaded with meaning. The monotony of my confined existence was inescapable. And once gestation was complete and my arachnid army was delivered, their principal mission was triggered: to manipulate every thought that entered my head.

Their first achievement was in hijacking my favourite number. As all children are acutely aware, it is of the utmost importance to have a favourite number, should you be asked by another young human what said favourite number happens to be. Mine had always been the number 16. The scorpions began to swarm around this number whenever it made an appearance. They drew my attention to it constantly, to its noble, dependable properties. It can be divided into 8s, 4s and 2s – all even, rounded numbers – which they assured me was a good thing. There is a smooth softness to the 6, a solid, anchoring foundation to the 1. But it was the 8s that interested me most, and I started to see them everywhere. Groupings of the number began to rise up and stand out against their backgrounds, as if illuminated by an unnatural sheen, daring me to look. The fingers on a pair of hands fascinated me, whilst the thumbs faded into soft focus. My eyes would seek out a constellation of eight small freckles on a stranger's arm. Each time the world around me filled me with fear, I heard the encouraging hum of the throng telling me to count. This silent counting kept the swelling panic at bay and became my own private barricade. At first it was the corners of rooms, the edges of mirrors, the frames of doorways.

1, 2, 3, 4, 5, 6, 7, 8

Each corner was gifted with its own dedicated count, whilst I stared – almost hypnotised – at the chosen nook. All eight numbers were given their due weight and time, before I moved on to the next 'unclean' corner, waiting to be baptised by my routine. To any unsuspecting person who witnessed this secret ritual in its infancy, it must have seemed that I was merely captivated by something unseen at the unremarkable intersection of household masonry that occurs in most rooms of a house – or that I had become, all of a sudden, lost in thought whilst my eyes came to rest upon the upper corners of whichever space I found myself in.

The looming threat of corners and edges soon became bigger, and the scorpions selected more perplexing enemies as obstacles to my daily routine:

pillows
curtains
TV screens
textbooks
light switches
pieces of toast

Everything needed to be counted, to be organised and contained by the number 8. If I didn't count, my protective little critters would thrash and stir, turning thoughts over and over until they span on one continuous loop. My blood would bubble and a feeling like a wave rising in a tsunami would build inside my chest, only to be stopped by the incessant counting.

So important did that counting become, that when I failed to carry out my instructed task, the scorpions planted darker thoughts to punish me for any noncompliance ...

If you don't finish the count,
your parents will die.

If you don't finish the count,
the house will burn down.

If you don't finish the count,
you will be sick.

Sickness was the threat most often used by the scorpions to shape my compulsive behaviour. Using still-vivid memories of my recent illness, they forged a fear like none I had ever known before. A fear of vomiting so acute that it was hard to think of almost anything else. My daily life was peppered with irrational musings.

If I consume this yoghurt after its 'use by' date
– I will vomit.

If I share this drink with anyone else
– I will vomit.

If I go to the local fair with my friends
– I will vomit.

So, by sticking to my silent counting rituals in order to quell the panic that surged in my chest, and by avoiding any situation that could possibly lead to my catching something or consuming something that would cause me to be sick, I managed to carry on with life in an outwardly normal fashion, all the while gratifying the guardians of my mind.

My secret remained as such until the night my mother discovered me on the landing, midway through one of my self-imposed routines. I explained to her the behaviours that I had to perform: the checking, the looking, the counting, and tried my best to tell her *why* I had to do each of these things, by which point I began to notice the expression that had taken hold of her face. She was listening to me in a way that children are not used to being listened to. Such focus and serious concern was she giving my protracted descriptions of what I now know to be compulsions, it made my own focus levels sharpen and I felt as though I was telling a secret that I had promised to keep private. Had I thought, or even noticed, that this behaviour was unusual – something peculiar for others to behold – I would have made more of a concerted effort to hide it. It was only by chance that my parents stumbled across these acts, easy as they were to perform discreetly; but until their untimely discovery, they had never been something that I had associated with shame. My scorpions had always been encouraging. Proud of my blind obedience. It was the consequent presence of doctors that made it all seem so aberrant. The more I began to feel I had betrayed them, the deeper the scorpions nestled in, stubborn in their attachment to those psychological burrows.

Following my parents' discovery of my routines, we once again visited our family doctor. He listened closely and sympathetically, quietly noting my attempts to under-play the effect of these routines on my daily life. Doctors' surgeries made me nervous and I was reluctant to admit to anything that would increase my attendance there. We agreed to keep an eye on the situation. To watch the scorpions as closely as they had been watching me. But, over the following months, they grew bigger and stron-ger, quicker and sneakier, and by my teenage years they had fully established themselves in my restive psyche. A part of the mental furniture. Therapy was naturally one of the first suggestions made by Dr G, but the idea of it scared me, making me feel like I had failed at the simple task of being normal. I didn't want to think there was something wrong with my mind, and I tried hard to hide the scorpions from my friends, allowing myself time to motor forward whilst I pretended to everyone around me that things were getting better. But, as my years at secondary school went by in a blur of arctic netball matches, broken hearts and a covertly hysterical love for Elvis Presley, I found myself once again at the door of our general practitioner's office. This time, although the symptoms were different from before, the solution he offered felt confrontingly medical.

'Have you thought about antidepressants?'

I exchanged a look of barely concealed terror with my mother, before reassuring him, 'I'm not depressed,

I just can't stop doing these routines. I don't want to take any tablets.'

Dr G's bedside manner adhered to that quintessential doctorly mix of utter kindness and cold, hard realism as he told me, 'It's actually very common that antidepressants are prescribed for your condition: they alter the way different parts of the brain communicate with each other, and the way in which obsessive compulsive disorder interrupts these processes.'

Obsessive-

Compulsive

Disorder.

It felt strange to hear it said aloud so flippantly. Until then we had largely referred to it as my 'routine'. The actual term was far too intimate, the way that he exposed the internal workings of my mind, and the words seemed to reverberate around the room, bouncing off each of the corners I was doing my very best not to count. It was too clinical. My nest of puppeteers in all their complexity reduced to scientific descriptors.

Something didn't feel quite right and I repeated, perhaps a little too strongly, 'I don't need any tablets,' to which he nodded and raised both hands in a defensive gesture.

'Fine. That's absolutely fine. But don't hesitate to come back and see me if you change your mind.'

And with that he handed me a pamphlet entitled 'Obsessive Compulsive Disorder: Help Is at Hand'. A menu of facts, statistics and unnervingly familiar case studies to peruse over dinner that evening.

On the short journey home, my mother and I agreed that it was the right decision to refuse the tablets. Medication was meant only for the severely mentally ill, the desperately unhappy or hardcore drug addicts – and I was coping just fine, we concurred. Everyone has their little quirks ...

Mental health was almost never talked about in our house – or any other house that we knew of, for that matter. There was nothing that I had ever seen, heard or read that correlated with my recent experience, and talking about it with anyone other than my parents or my doctor would have felt akin to peeling off several layers of skin and standing naked in the school playground at the height of winter. It remained an unexplored taboo, best kept where it belonged – under hats and behind closed doors.

As I crept towards the end of my school days, I managed the scorpions relatively well. I allowed one or two new routines to slip through the net in order to keep them quiet in my more stressful moments. One involved counting the drips falling from the bathroom tap after turning it off; another revolved around touching the knobs of the gas cooker eight times before leaving the house – but there was nothing that anyone aside from my family would have noticed. After all, the limited information to be found on the earliest incarnation of the internet (the one that assaulted your eardrums for twenty seconds with a high-frequency scream in exchange for accessing it) told me that 1 in 50 people lived with their own scorpions, so I was just another anonymous member of this little club. They remained stimulated, sated and, most importantly, almost entirely secret. Of course, it was in their interest to remain secret – they didn't want anyone trying to get rid of them – which meant that they were at their most alert when I was at home. At school they could be humiliated or forced into the light; at home they felt free in their familiar spaces.

The abject terror that the idea of vomiting induced in my body was constant background music, especially in an institution populated by children whose immune systems were yet to find their adult levels of stability, but the compulsions themselves would suffer at the hands of distraction, and I was able to forget about them for long periods of the day whilst I was at school. I later realised that my OCD and the routines that came with it were intertwined with a sense of responsibility. At school the property, the classrooms, the playground were not my responsibility to maintain or watch over. I could leave a classroom at school without counting the corners each time because there were thirty other children and a teacher inside the room who also shared that space, so if I were to leave and the room was to burn to the ground or something bad was to happen, I could convince myself that I wasn't carrying sole responsibility for that negative outcome. The same logic did not seem to apply at home, perhaps due to the fact that much of my time with ME/ CFS was spent indoors, in my room, so I felt a sense of duty to keep that house and all of its inhabitants safe. It was my castle, the place where everyone I loved most in the world, slept and ate and *lived*.

By Sixth Form, an extracurricular passion for theatre slowly began to filter into my school life. I had always been hungry for hobbies, but often found myself getting bored too quickly, or becoming furious that I hadn't immediately become a prodigy at whatever craft or skill I was attempting to learn. This resulted in my ardently investing in and then abruptly discarding a variety of different after-school courses or classes, until I finally hit upon a local theatre group in which I, miraculously, seemed to maintain some interest. Before long, I was signing up to every school play, every performance, every assembly reading, and to my utter surprise, I didn't seem to care how rubbish I was. As my school years drew to an end and decisions about the future loomed, it became obvious to me, and probably my teachers, that there was nothing besides acting that I really wanted to do. The careers advisor assigned to our class was evidently troubled by my choice of university application.

'Oh, right. But a drama school isn't really a *real* university, is it?' said Mrs P, pronouncing the words 'drama' and 'school' with the most peculiar intonation, as if their sitting next to each other constructed an entirely alien concept.

'Well, I don't want to go to university. I want to be an actress.' My response reignited the look of bewilderment she had been suppressing throughout our session, and she tried again to convert me to one of the more favourable career paths encouraged by the school, despite my obvious lack of credentials to pursue any of them.

'If you apply to university, you could study English, or perhaps law – that requires a certain flair for drama. Or even journalism? Theatre studies can be a useful foundation for all of these subjects, and that way you can have a solid Plan B!'

I was quietly seething at the idea of having a Plan B, and felt a crawling sensation start to envelop my brain. One of the many things, good and bad, that my ME/CFS had given me was the power to daydream. Long stretches of time alone confined to my bed allowed for the perfect conditions in which imagination could take flight. I became the carved wooden puppet serenaded so sweetly by a uniform-clad Elvis in *G.I. Blues*. I was the lone-wolf investigator searching for patterns linking serial killers in the gruesome book of case studies that I begged my parents to buy me for my sixteenth birthday. In *The NeverEnding Story*, I was Atreyu walking anxiously towards the laser-eyed guardians of the Sphinx Gate.

So, against the better judgement of Mrs P, but with the full support of my parents, I applied to study acting at drama school and arrived at a crossroads in my young life. I was ready to escape the familiar clutches of my forceful beasts and make sure that they moved out of their home at the same time as I moved out of mine. It should have been easy enough. All I had to do was stop doing my routines. A change of environment would surely suffice to show them the door. As long as I stopped counting and touching and didn't invent any new rituals for each room of my student digs, then I would be fine. They would leave me alone and I could get on with the daunting task of becoming an adult, just like everyone else. And so, consumed by a desire to take back control, I finally said goodbye to the little town I'd never thought I'd leave and readied myself to banish the scorpions for good. But as I finished packing up my life for London and buckled myself into the back seat of our family car, my parents chattering excitedly about the year ahead, a fable I once read was stuck on a loop in my mind:

A scorpion wants to cross a river but it cannot swim, so it asks a frog sitting on the bank to carry it to the other side. The frog hesitates, afraid that the scorpion might sting. The scorpion argues that if it did so, the frog would die and they would both drown. After considering this argument, the frog agrees to ferry the scorpion across. As they approach the midpoint of the river, the scorpion stings the frog, dooming them both. The dying frog asks the scorpion why it chose to sting despite knowing the fatal consequences, to which the scorpion replies: 'I couldn't help it. It's in my nature.'

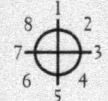

BEDROOM RITUAL

☒   Stand with your toes touching bedroom doorway.
Lights off.

☒   Push the door open with both hands resting on either
side of the handle.

☒   Locate the four corners of the room.

☒   Starting with the closest corner on the left, look directly
at it and begin to count:

1, 2, 3, 4, 5, 6, 7, 8.

☒   If you take your eyes off the corner, you must start the
count again.

☒   Once finished, move one corner to the right and start
again.

☒   Only move on to the next corner once fully satisfied.*

☒   From left to right, check all four corners, counting 1 to 8
for each.

☒   Repeat the cycle for each corner, so every one has it's
turn as the new 'starter' corner. Repeat until you reach
the one to the right of where you started.

*Satisfaction occurs only when the anxiety stops and the
tightness in the chest diminishes.*

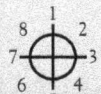

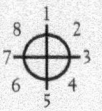

☒   Begin the entire cycle again, but this time going backwards from right to left. Repeat for four rounds.

☒   Repeat counts of 1 to 8 moving both clockwise and anticlockwise, on each of the corners of your room and the following square or rectangular objects:

> *mirror*
> *bed*
> *poster*
> *television screen*
> *cupboard doors*
> *rug*
> *bookshelf*
> *window.*

☒   When the cycle is finished for each corner, switch on the lights and repeat again for every object, beginning as before with the corners of the room.

☒   Once complete, the bedroom can be entered.

☒   Finally, to sleep soundly, count the corners of the duvet once in bed.

☒   (NB: Routine must be carried out in silence and with as little movement as possible, so as not to alert others to the presence of the scorpions.)

Chapter Two

MATING/
RITUALS

'Scorpions are solitary animals that avoid
each other to reduce the risk of cannibalism.'

Gary A. Polis et al., 'Predators of Scorpions'

With a gun to my head I couldn't tell you if it's sweat or tears I can feel trickling down in salty rivulets over my flushed cheeks and pooling uncomfortably in the shallow hollow beneath my throat. It is an unseasonably hot September day in London, I am eighteen years old, and am being forced to do more exercise than I ever thought possible. Four days into my first week of drama school, our class is partaking in what's been termed a 'Shakedown' by our physical theatre tutor, Mr F, and which can only be described as a mix between military bootcamp and a drug-less hardcore rave. We are all wildly unprepared. Several of the girls have forgotten hairbands, drenched locks plastered to their necks, and up until now the concept of sportswear has been altogether lost on me. I am wearing a kind of loose linen smock and dancing in bare feet, not only because my footwear is unsuitable but because it's really too hot to be wearing anything at all. The room is several storeys up with windows stretching its entire length, and the afternoon sun is beating in through the glass panes, making us feel like we are peering through an oven door out on to the outside world, where air moves freely and one's free will remains intact. There are varying levels of fitness on display in our group, but none can match the endurance of Mr F, who – one and a half hours in – continues to pump his sinewy arms to the beat without breaking a sweat, switching effortlessly between rhythmic shamanic dance and a kind of choreographed shadow-boxing. He is lean, hairless, impressively aerodynamic, and at this moment appears to be on an entirely different planet. I am not lucky enough to have transcended into that other, allegedly pleasurable, realm experienced only within the upper echelons of athletic euphoria, but my body has instead stayed firmly tethered to a reality in which my muscles sting, my head is spinning and the floor is – quite literally – lava. My eyes flick to the clock for the 400th time since the session began and I am crushed to discover we have another half an hour left of this purgatory. The only 'rules' of the Shakedown are that you must not stop moving and you are not allowed to speak. The purpose of the exercise is to awaken our bodies and communicate through physical expression alone. You can use the space, the floor, the walls, the mirrors as you wish, but you cannot stop moving as long as the music is playing. The heat is punishing, so I decide to buy myself a few seconds rest by 'using' the floor, rolling slowly from side to side and jutting my legs into the air lamely at acceptable intervals. I look like a dying insect. I snatch a look at Mr F to ensure that I haven't been caught, and although his eyes are shooting laser beams of pure, unadulterated enthusiasm into the room, I am pretty sure he isn't experiencing sight through either one of them. The music shifts into a new dimension and his limbs lock briefly into a demented tableau as he lets rip another Wembley Arena-sized: *'DON'T. STOP. MOOOOOVING!'*

I am yet to make any friends after almost a week, despite my careful observation of the group, but am thrilled to find this collective form of dance-torture is bringing out the more playful side of my classmates. One girl in particular has caught my attention. She has a sort of bouncy, hysterical gait and a contagiously knowing smirk that plays on her lips each time we lock eyes across the room. I see her springy brown curls bounding towards me as she discovers my attempt to slack off, and she too dives to the floor with a show of mock creativity. Like me, she is desperate to break the talking rule and shatter this circus of earnestness, but keeps losing her nerve and instead tries to communicate her discomfort through wide-eyed stares and farcical hand gestures. We both descend into silent fits of giggling.

This ritualistic dance persists on a repeated loop as we continue to find each other amongst the sea of melting bodies, assessing one another as new potential mates. As the minute hand thunks into place, finally signalling the end of the class, I can see her shiny smiling face fill my peripheral vision and she approaches me with an enviable ease. I am so out of breath I can barely form a sentence.

'Hey,' is her opener. A warm Yorkshire twang cuddles the word.

'Hey,' I counter, wheezingly.

She pushes an escaped ringlet back off her forehead. 'Can I have some of your water?'

I look down at my hands clutching a plastic two-litre bottle of the good stuff, unsure quite how to play my next move. The bottle is almost full due to the fact that I only really started drinking water six months ago and am still trying my best to pretend that I like it. It is no less than a miracle that I appear to have survived into my late teens having largely consumed just tea, orange squash and strawberry Ribena to maintain basic levels of hydration.

'No. Sorry.'

She laughs. An open, friendly cackle which dies as quickly as it started when she sees the look of sincerity fixed upon my face. 'No?'

'Sorry. I don't share drinks,' I explain, baring my teeth apologetically.

Her face drops. 'Oh, OK ... Cool.' She is sweating profusely and drifts away in search of a kinder human being to help keep her alive in her moment of need. I consider following but decide against it, too exhausted to offer up an explanation for my total lack of generosity or care. I stand by and watch as she gulps unselfconsciously from my neighbour's appetising flagon. They chat like old friends, and every now and then, as I pack up my bag to go home, I can hear her cackle ring out across the room, the underscore to yet another meet-cute I have unintentionally ruined. Untouched water bottle in hand, I scurry shamefully out of the room, passing the teeming student bar on my way, to go home and think about what I've done.

Then think about it again.

And again.

And again.

As luck would have it, this Northern angel was completely unfazed by my introductory rudeness. Over the months that followed, we found in each other a kindred spirit. We shared the same dark humour, a mutually idiotic decision to abstain from alcohol for the entire three years of training (for reasons neither of us can remember to this day), and a capacity to remember the most obscure and ultimately useless details about every person we ever met. Rather than reject my often antisocial behaviour, she understood and even made light of what I had previously considered to be my strangeness. Despite a potentially rocky start, I had successfully made a new friend.

In my experience, OCD thrives in solitude, making intimate childhood friendships something of a minefield. All the things that are designed to help us strengthen bonds with other children were all things that I resolutely avoided. Group gatherings, sleepovers, school trips. One evening, after daring to accept a weekend invitation to a new schoolfriend's house for dinner, I returned home to greet my mother with a stomach full of knots and a pocket full of onion rings. I had been convinced that the onions were somehow undercooked inside their battered coats, turning each into a little Petri dish of bacteria, and so with my nimble twelve-year-old fingers hidden below the dining-room table, I had extracted each ribbon of onion from its circular tunnel and laid them flat in my napkin, before squirrelling them away in my school blazer, to be disposed of several hours later, all the while managing to uphold polite levels of conversation with the unsuspecting family who were hosting me. Dinner invitations at friends' houses with their exhausting glut of unknowns became too much for my fuddled mind to negotiate, and so I avoided them. I felt overwhelmed by big groups and paralysed by the fear that if I were to risk enjoying myself by partaking in a night or two away from home then I would be struck down by a virus that might make me vomit in the unfamiliar toilet of an unfamiliar home and find myself beyond the reach of my parents' mysterious healing powers. So, at my own insistence, I missed out on many social gatherings throughout my teenage years that most other people might have billed as 'fun'.

I still observe large friendship groups like a detached cat watching a swarm of bees. At times watching nervously from an acceptable distance, at others coming in too excited or heavy-handed and smashing every opportunity for progress dead, but all the while knowing that I have always ultimately felt like a different species. One of the solitary ones. Something in my DNA, in the ancient make-up of mankind, understands that this makes no sense. Humans are pack animals; we need others to survive. Yet the warm embrace of the masses sends me running for the hills. I don't honestly know whether OCD has fuelled my love of solitude or whether seeking solitude allowed my OCD to blossom, but whichever statement is the truth, I have come to realise that as an adult it is something I find absolutely necessary to help me reset in times of stress or anxiety. The environment around me has a very clear and direct effect on how I am able to cope when the world is moving just a little too fast. Besides, faced with the demoralising task of presenting myself to the world as an agreeable sort of friend, I have often fallen at the first hurdle.

When I explain to somebody new that I have OCD, I have found the majority of people to be understanding and supportive, but there still seems to be a disconnect in the way some people receive the actual reality of specific obsessive thought patterns. Almost everyone immediately accepts my aversion to bacteria and need for cleanliness without a second thought, but it is pretty commonplace for me to inadvertently offend someone with my vomiting phobia. Although they understand what I am telling them and I have informed them that it is an illogical phobia and not a personal judgement against them, I have lost count of the times that I have had to apologise repeatedly to a sceptical and wounded acquaintance or colleague when avoiding physical contact or even being in the same room as them after learning they have been vomiting (or have been in close contact with someone who has). I once succeeded in alienating my personal dresser on a theatre production, by grilling her so extensively about her admission to having vomited until 3am the previous night, that she chose not to dress me for the remainder of the play, and not only avoided me in the many labyrinthine corridors of the building, but never made eye contact with me again. Then again, at the age of thirty-two, I managed to derail my own book club by drafting a fairly militant set of ground rules and insisting upon impossible levels of commitment from the members (a lovely, free-spirited group of women), resulting in the club ultimately disbanding and my attempts to create the larger friendship group I'd always felt I was supposed to have failing spectacularly.

Relationships with an OCD person can be a complex affair too. Presenting a relatively sane expression of yourself to the world can backfire when navigating the subsequent period of 'getting to know' one another. The compulsions can no longer be hidden, the thoughts can't be held at bay when you are sharing your space with another thinking, feeling human being every hour of the day. I am often reminded of the way female scorpions devour their mates after copulation. Perhaps they are never really *intending* to eat them? It is just easier that way.

The art of obsessing needs time and space, both of which are at their most plenteous in the absence of other people. This need to be alone, however, is somewhat at odds with the fact that my obsessive mind never likes *other things* to be alone. If I drop a crisp on the floor by accident, rendering it too dirty to eat, I will either drop another, so that it is not on its own, or split the existing crisp into two so that there are an even number of crisps on the floor. I don't want that crisp to feel lonely. Similarly, I once transformed a daily commute via the same familiar footpath into a fraught one, obsessed by the fact that I had dropped one of my hairclips on the ground without realising. I would pass this dropped hairclip every day, wracked with guilt but unable to save it from a future of solitude and filth. It was partially covered with a sort of shiny liquid that I couldn't identify, and so I left it there, alone, and put my best efforts into ignoring both the clip itself and the bubble of shame that rose up in my gut each time I passed it by. This is not only because my strand of OCD favours *even* numbers, but also because since I was very young I have awarded all inanimate objects with human feelings. I was far older than I'd care to admit when I finally managed to dispose of a dog that I had lovingly made out of a discarded cereal box. I still feel guilty when I think of it, pulped or disintegrated, outside in the cold, no other cardboard dogs for companionship ...

When I left home for London at the beginning of my journey through drama school, I knew that for the first time I would be living with people other than members of my own family, and the idea unnerved me. Would I still feel the need to do my routines once my environment had changed? Would I be able to hide my compulsions around my new housemates? Did I *want* to hide them?

I had opted to live with three young men during my first year, selected from a list shared by the school of other students who were also looking to flat-share. Two excitable best friends from Middlesborough, who communicated 55 per cent of the time through song, and an elusive kung-fu champion who imprisoned himself in his tiny room for hours on end, either listening to Franz Liszt and quoting Laurence Olivier at equally impressive volumes or playing *Tekken* 3 on a television screen he had balanced at almost ceiling height atop an enormous wooden wardrobe. Having experienced a tricky female friendship triangle at the beginning of primary school, I felt safe with the boys. To cohabit with this new unlikely trio felt strangely uncomplicated. I had hoped that the distraction of a disciplined daily schedule, the constant presence of new personalities, and residing in an apartment for which I shared only a quarter of the responsibility might rid me of my compulsive rituals for good. I had hoped that it was habit born of a time and place that I had now left behind. However, the routines travelled with me. Tucked into my pockets, weighing me down like a soggy napkin full of onion rings.

The routines developed. They became longer and more complex, which often made me late leaving the house. Late attendance to our course was tolerated on a 'three strikes and you're out' basis, so there was a particularly all-consuming kind of pressure that accompanied my ritualistic checking in the first year of training. When rushed or working against a fixed deadline, my anxiety over having to complete a routine quickly naturally increased, so my focus scattered and I had to repeat the routine more times than usual before I could leave the house satisfied.

My routines or compulsions centre (and have always centered) around two main points of focus: home environment and illness/death. Both categories are inflamed by stress or anxiety, and both remain a constant fascination for the scorpions. Whether my home is a permanent or a temporary one, there are certain areas within that familiar space that become an obstacle to my ability to function normally. It is *leaving* the house that presents me with the biggest challenge. A typical thought/behaviour cycle I experience often as an adult will go something like this:

> *I'm standing in the middle of my kitchen and am already ten minutes late.* **But if I perform the routine one more time, then this feeling of impending <u>doom</u> might just go away long enough for me to get out the front door.** I hold my hand palm up beneath the tap, staring at the empty space where running water would usually flow. **<u>It's definitely off.</u>** *However, despite the fact that I have a pair of fully functioning eyes and my logical brain tells me that there is no water touching my hand,* I cannot seem to accept this reality as true. *Can I feel the water?* **<u>NO</u>**.

Can I see it? **NO**.

Can I hear it?

I close my eyes for a moment and take a deep breath, listening for the gentle hiss and splash that *never comes.*

I open my eyes again and everything remains the same, not least my belief that somehow the tap is still running at full flow into the sink. **I press my thumb onto the closed faucet, trace the contours of the metal, committing its physicality to memory.**

I look. I count. I've lost track of the minutes I've been standing here.

I move to the cooker. **The gas is off.** <u>*I know it's off.*</u> But gas is invisible, so how do I know it isn't slowly leaking into every room of my house and I won't die of suffocation in my sleep later tonight? *Or, when I forget this whole charade and next decide to light a candle, might I* **ignite my own death** *with the flick of a match? I begin to imagine a scene several hours later in which an enormous house fire destroys all my belongings, kills my cat, and spreads rapidly through my neighbours' houses, turning the entire street into a pile of dust and ashes.*

The thoughts soon become more abstract, and I feel completely out of control of the vast number of scenarios that could occur if I fail to stay on my guard.

If there is a type of cancer that I don't know the symptoms for, then that will be the cancer that kills me. If I don't step onto the centre of those four consecutive paving slabs whilst walking, the next plane a loved one gets on will crash. (Even committing that last sentence to the page was a special type of agony. My desire to be honest about my intrusive thoughts versus the abject fear of bringing them to fruition through mere utterance or acknowledgement of the idea is an ever-present conflict.)

In the midst of these thought cycles, I might send a quick message to my agent/friend/family member to say I am running late. Transport issues, I'd say. Now I would have to start my routine again. The message would break my cycle of concentration and it is as if my short-term memory has been instantaneously erased. I'd put my bag down defeatedly and start my mental count as I look at the various enemies occupying my kitchen: door, tap, cooker, fridge, light switch.

I'd promise myself this was the last time. After all, I'd still have more rooms to check before I could leave.

1,2,3,4,5,6,7,8.
1,2,3,4,5,6,7,8.

The counting happens almost without thought or intention now. It is so ingrained, so practised, that I can perform it in a kind of standby mode. The scorpions take over, so I don't have to think. I can have a conversation, carry out tasks simultaneously and entertain entirely new thoughts as the numbers tick over in my brain. They are a place-holder for reassurance. The repetition soothes me like a mantra, giving me time to breathe and order my thoughts, but they have also become a type of code. The emotional pressure I feel building in my chest before I have finished the count is akin to the experience of watching the cock-sure young antihero in a nail-biting thriller try to crack the criminal's safe, whilst the owner of the jewels/money/documents makes their way up the stairs towards them with only seconds to spare before we can finally breathe a sigh of relief and our hero escapes. If I count enough times and I crack the code to the safe, I stop something bad from happening. The house won't flood. The cat won't die. My family won't be hurt. I won't get sick. That's the bargain I strike with the scorpions. It is not always possible to achieve a satisfactory outcome when perform-ing routines, and I am frequently left feeling even more anxious, which adds fuel to an already-roaring fire. If I still feel unable to move on from the routine I am stuck on, I have begun to rely on a fairly simple coping mechanism: taking photographs. I have an online photo album that is forever in a state of full capacity due to the excess of mundane domestic photography I insist on housing there. I take and keep photographs of doors, ovens, locks, fridges, windows, lamps, candles and plug sockets, with the sole purpose of calming my anxious future mind. If I have left the house and no longer trust my prior assessment of the various obstacles that have been plotting to ruin my day, then I can look at the photograph I took at the time of the ritual to reassure myself that the oven is in fact off, the door is in fact shut and the candles are in fact unlit. I have more photographs of doors on my phone than I have of my friends.

It so happens (or I suppose that it is not in any small way a coincidence) that many of my friends are also in some way neurodiverse. There is, of course, a wide spectrum, and the entire population exists somewhere along that spectrum, but for me it has been a relief to know that I have support and understanding from friends who know first-hand what I might be experiencing. Naturally I have unlimited reserves of sympathy for anyone carrying scorpions of their own, but there is a delicate balance at play, as hearing about the rituals and compulsions that others are compelled to partake in sometimes presents me with a problem. How do I shut off the part of my brain that immediately wants to adopt these compulsions as my own? How can I close the door on the scorpions? It is a choice between being a good friend and inheriting another compulsion to add to my already-stretched repertoire of rituals or fighting my gut to protect myself and displaying a perceived lack of compassion by shutting my ears to another's individual struggles. I am constantly battling with my desire to be a valuable friend, partner or colleague, whilst keeping the most challenging sides of my OCD at bay. If a plan changes from what was originally agreed, I find it hard to accept. If a loved one is ill and they need to be taken care of, I am not there – for fear of catching something. If a friend is cooking me a meal and I am suspicious of the use-by date of one of the ingredients, I will interrogate them to the point of ruining their gesture of kindness. I hate these things about myself, but often feel powerless to change them.

After my drama-school training it became obvious that three years is not long enough to *learn* how to become an actor. You spend your entire career learning, as you spend your entire life learning how to become a human being. Each year of my training I learned new skills, new processes, but I also learned how to pretend beyond the confines of acting. To pretend I was calm or composed. That there wasn't a nest of scorpions living inside my brain. It is an exhausting way to function, to constantly hide a part of yourself that is so intrinsic and unappealing. I have no doubt that I am a better pretender than I am an actor, so adept at moving through life undetected that I can almost convince *myself* that the scorpions are not there.

But they are there. Meddling, goading, rewarding. So what could be a better defence against the scorpions than to make friends with them? A friendship that, if I think about it, has long preceded most of my human ones. Surely that alone is something worth hiding?

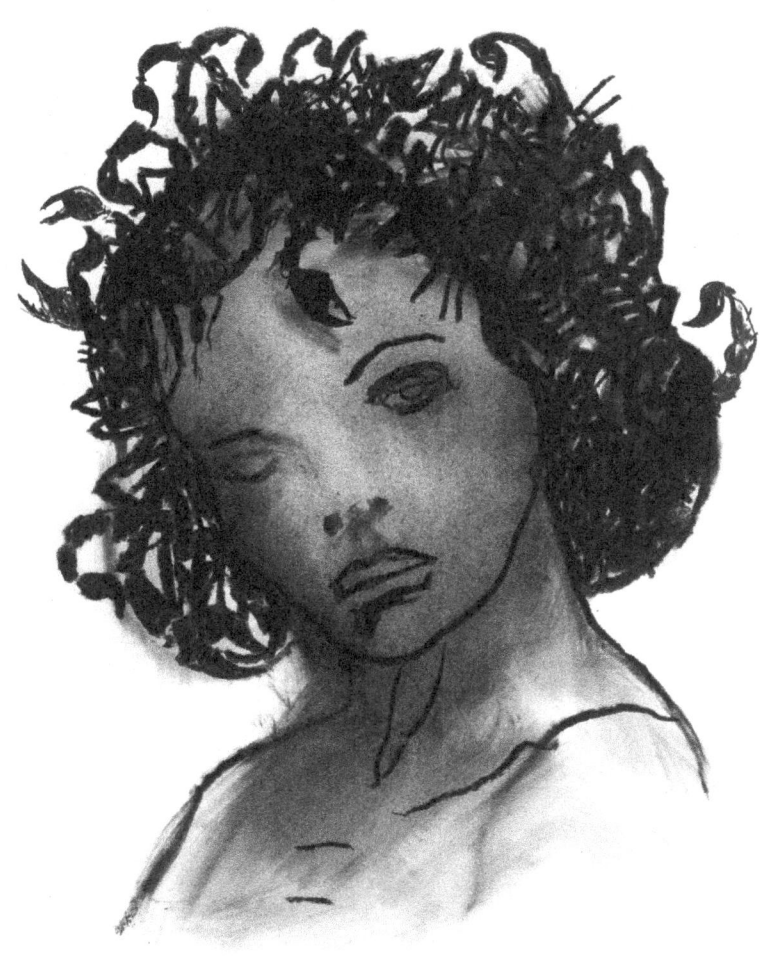

Sedusa; misconceived

Chapter Three

VOMIT

'Scorpions as organisms with relatively long lifespans
are more likely to be exposed to a pathogen multiple
times during their lifetime; therefore, they are good
candidates to show immune priming.'

Dumas Gálvez et al., 'Immune priming against bacteria
in spiders and scorpions?'

The sun is low as I ascend the steps to the aeroplane and turn back, squinting into the dusky orange light to say a silent goodbye to the beautiful city of Prague. I have the same feeling I always have when leaving a filming project behind, a sort of pleasant melancholy bubbling away in the pit of my stomach. I remain conflicted, however, as to the benefits of an evening flight. On the one hand I am treated to a full final day in my temporary homeland, a peaceful and solitary farewell to another chapter of my life; but on the other, it affords excess time for my particular anxiety to take root. More time allows for more space in which to house this litany of home-grown terrors, and, as always, the journey begins long before I catch sight of the plane.

It is more than a decade since I left drama school, but I still cannot shake the nervousness I feel at having to travel for work. By that I don't mean the changing environments or the new people, but simply the act of using a mode of transport, particularly planes, to get there. Yet here I am again. The queue to board the plane back to London is moving at a snail's pace and I can feel my thoughts in freefall, my busy little critters at their most alert. I close my eyes and breathe deeply. Try to align their speed of movement with that of the meandering passengers ahead. As I approach the door to the aircraft, my right hand hovers in the air, attached by invisible strings to many tiny pairs of pincers, manoeuvring it towards the top edge of the doorframe. I am no longer in control of my body and my fingers tap twice on the cool metal, unseen by the other passengers, as I wait to be greeted by an impossibly friendly air steward wearing red-rimmed glasses that perfectly frame his red-rimmed eyes.

I borrowed this particular ritual from a friend who once told me his only tendency towards superstition was to tap the outside of the aeroplane before every flight he boarded 'to keep him safe'. I laughed along at the time, but the moment the confession left his lips, I had taken the idea hostage in my brain. I had only intended to try it out, perhaps once or twice when I next flew somewhere, but then my scorpions developed a predictable attachment to this new offering, and so it became that the loan was a permanent one.

Once inside the plane, the activity ramps up a notch and my darlings have placed me on high alert. I search for my row number and exhale relief as I realise I have secured the coveted window seat, an illusion that I am still connected to the outside world. An escape, albeit small, from the curved walls of the aircraft that form the flying prison in which I have just willingly detained myself.

One of the perks of travelling to or from a film location shoot is that the production will often fly their actors business class. Something I relish not for the free miniatures and microwaved ready-meals, but the guaranteed *space* between you and the person next to you. A luxurious foot and a half from potential infection. It is not the 36,000 feet that I fear when flying, or the horrifying certainty of death if faced with a catastrophic engine failure. It is something that remains fairly low on most people's lists of anxieties when jetting off on holiday or conducting a business trip ... I find myself smiling a little too keenly and much too frequently at the flow of people passing me by, to give an impression of exceptional calm at being trapped aboard a gigantic metal incubator with them for the best part of two hours. No one smiles back. Perhaps they think I am afraid of flying?

They would be wrong. The thing that terrifies me is *vomit*.

To my mind, there are only two types of vomit: GOOD VOMIT and BAD VOMIT. In order to help you distinguish between these categories, I have provided a conclusive list:

GOOD VOMIT
The milky spittle of a newborn baby
Projectiles born of food poisoning

Drunken purging
Hung-over purging
Motion sickness (regardless of transport type)
Morning sickness

BAD VOMIT
The product of all varieties of infectious viral or
bacterial illnesses, e.g. norovirus and its many grisly
associates

Of course, to be the victim of the majority of the entries on both lists is a miserable ordeal for anyone (and for my particular kind of OCD, to throw up in any context is a disaster of epic proportions which must be avoided at all costs), but when encountering other people suffering from the affliction it is the culprits on the BAD VOMIT list who send me into a cold sweat. The obvious difference being that you cannot *catch* the causes of sickness on the former list, and so they become relatively harmless (yet disgusting) little inconveniences when performed by those in one's immediate vicinity.

Back on the plane, my trusty routine is triggered by the toughened black crusaders living inside me, and I am subjected to a ballet of intrusive thoughts. It begins with scanning. My inane smiling is really just a mask for my true mission: to carefully assess each of the other passengers for signs of illness or fatigue. This proves to be an infuriating task, as it is not uncommon for the average person to feel a little tired, neurotic or groggy on a plane journey, therefore appearing somewhat out of sorts – and it makes my assessment much more complicated. Is that woman three rows behind me falling asleep because she has recently caught a vomiting bug, which has not yet presented its symptoms but has been incubating for the last twenty-four hours in her unsuspecting immune system, therefore making her sleep in order to prepare her for the hideous onslaught that is surely due to make an appearance in the next hour or so, exposing me and the other passengers to her unavoidable contagion? Is that gentle rustling at the very front of the plane the sound of someone reaching for their complimentary sick bag, ready to unleash hell just as the 'fasten seatbelt' signs light up and render me captive for the entire journey? And why is that man using the toilet only moments after locating his seat? It can only be ascribed to the fact that his uncontrollable urge to vomit has forced him to push back against the flow of traffic entering the plane to distribute the many millions of infectious airborne micro-particles generously inside the confined space of the aircraft loo.

It is important to reference that at this point, the research that I have been encouraged to do over the decades by my devoted arthropods comes into play quite heavily. They are not foolish creatures, and they thrive on evidence for their claims, so it has always been essential to provide proof to back up each one of my fears. If someone tells me they have vomited and that they 'think' it was something they ate, I will categorically not believe them unless I see a hand-signed note from a hospital declaring as much. Similarly, if I am told that 'you can't catch a virus from the air', I am inclined to require evidence to confirm this. One of the more scientific nuggets I have found to bolster my ever-expanding case was sourced from the scientific journal *PLOS One* and states that 'when one person vomits, the aerosolised virus particles can get into another person's mouth and, if swallowed, can lead to infection'.

AEROSOLISED.

The conclusion being, there is no escape. That is unless society's collective daily aim is to avoid catching norovirus at all costs, which – in my opinion – it absolutely should be.

One of the signature features of an obsessive intrusive thought cycle is that they are rarely, if ever, influenced by fact. But like a good lie, which invariably includes a modicum of truth, an obsessive thought cycle is often laced with elements of logic, however weak or persuasive they might be. In 2014 Dr Catherine Makison Booth wrote an article for the *Journal of Infection Prevention* (where do I subscribe?) about her invention, 'Vomiting Larry' – a simulated vomiting machine created to assess environmental contamination from projectile vomiting related to norovirus infection. She cites that there can be 'as many as a thousand million viruses in the vomit and diarrhoea produced by infected individuals, yet it takes only 10 to 100 viruses to cause infection in the next unaffected person'. Using UV light and water seeded with a fluorescent dye in her man-made vomiting system, Dr Makison Booth's team has shown that droplets of 'vomited' fluid can cover an area in excess of 7.8 metres. Alongside this, she concluded that virus particles will wait happily in any given environment for weeks or longer, resisting most active ingredients in cleaning products. These particles, if transferred to someone's hands, can be transmitted to another person who touches them. If it gets into the air, the virus can land in another person's mouth and infect them that way. Contaminated food is also a common transmission route, usually as a result of food workers not washing their hands sufficiently. And, to top it all off, a person who feels better after a few days may still be shedding the virus for many more, so can spread it to others whilst appearing entirely recovered themselves. Noroviruses are diverse, and so even if your immune system learns to fight off one, it'll likely be helpless against other future iterations.

So, all things considered, it's a living fucking nightmare.

'Doors to manual and cross-check.'

I tune back in to a hum of chatter and metallic clunks as the aeroplane is sealed shut and I realise that I have won the aviation lottery. The two seats next to me are free and I have the entire row to myself. I cannot believe my luck. My preliminary scan of the passengers has been a successful one, no signs of suspicious behaviour or pallid complexions, and the prospect of breathing the same recycled air as 150 strangers for two hours suddenly feels a little less frightening. I settle in to my chair and look out across the tarmac, my eyes following a cartoonish miniature lorry pulling a caterpillar of wobbly suitcases towards the gaping mouth of an aeroplane hold. I am jealous of those suitcases, huddled beneath a congregation of living, breathing holidaymakers, exempt from the agony of small talk and potential cross-contamination. How I wish to be a little sedated dog, holed up between that mountain of bags, transported from A to B in a blur of unpeopled vignettes.

I perform the final practices that will assure my safe delivery to my destination unharmed: eating a Werther's Original and rereading a text from my mother that says 'Safe flight darling' a minimum of four times, before sliding my phone into airplane mode and glaring spinelessly at others who don't. The engines rumble and we soar into the air, a collective breath held, and whilst those first precious seconds tick by, I listen closely for disconcerting clangs, urgent whispers, and tinny, distant pleas of 'Mayday! Mayday!'

I allow my eyes to close as the momentary silence gives way to a cacophony of nervous laughter and idle conversation.

There is a coughing sound to my left. My head snaps instantaneously towards the sound and a stampede is triggered. This time it does not happen slowly; my scorpions are prepared and have chosen to send the full battalion to the front line – there is no time to lose.

The perpetrator is a man in his mid-forties. He is sitting in the window seat directly across from mine, and he too has managed to secure a row all to himself, so I have a perfect, uninterrupted view of the action unfolding. He is hunched over, facing the window, and I watch in terror as his back arches violently, a guttural growl escaping his body. My pulse quickens and I begin to feel a familiar desert heat rushing to my palms when he turns a few degrees to the right and I see what his body has been concealing. In his hands, pale and shaking, he grips the edges of a crumpled white sick bag, straining beneath the weight of its innards. Or, more accurately, his innards. The first deluge of questions floods my mind as the scorpions rush to my defence. *How did I miss this? How long has he been vomiting? Why was he allowed on the plane?* The barricade has begun, and my home-grown army works at triple speed to stop any infectious particles boarding my system and hijacking its fertile breeding ground. Without thinking, my arms reach for the scarf bundled beneath my chair and I loop it twice around my neck – a little too tight, to constrict my breathing – then with the remaining length I completely cover my mouth, nose and the top of my head, leaving only a narrow window slicing across both eyes, the only means through which I can view my own personalised horror film. The scorpions lie heavy on my chest, and my breathing becomes quicker and lighter. I wish for a moment that I could hold my breath entirely, that I could stop gulping this virulent air, but a panic takes hold that I cannot override. Each exhale is more violent than the last, as if thrusting the air from my lungs will clear any germs that might have settled in the soft, moist tissue inside my mouth and nasal cavities. The combination of these reverse gut-punches and the small, shallow sips of oxygen I reluctantly allow myself are making me lightheaded, and I feel a thumping sensation as the blood rushes to my head, cheeks burning against the heat of my woollen helmet.

'Would you like any drinks, madam?' smiles Red-Rimmed Glasses, who has appeared from nowhere and has clearly chosen to ignore my choice of improvised head-wear. Another retch rings out, followed by the dull splash of vomit on vomit. The sound travels through me like a gunshot and I look at the steward with the terrified eyes of a hunted antelope peering through thick Saharan grass.

'Is – is he OK?' I stammer. 'Why is he being sick?' Red-Rimmed Glasses throws a casual look over his shoulder, apparently unaware of the grotesque spectacle occurring just a few feet behind him.

'Uhh, I'm not sure. Did you want any drinks, or … ?'

To me, it is an entirely dumbfounding notion that other people do not spend a significant portion of each day analysing or fretting about the various ways in which anyone and everyone around them could be infectiously sick. Any other illness is child's play as far as I am concerned. I will happily remain in close contact with a common cold or the full spectrum of contagious skin conditions. But I am baffled anew when faced with yet another scorpion-less individual who not only *doesn't* think about vomit fourteen hours a day, but is completely unfazed by an actively vomiting person sitting at such dangerously close range that you can practically feel several thousand viral particles clinging to the air around your mouth, waiting to be invited in on the next inevitable intake of breath.

'No. No drinks. He's sick. Maybe ask why?' I am trying to use as few words as possible. Every word means a longer sentence, which means more breath is required of me, and I am not risking taking more breaths than I need to. The effect is a strange one. I am simultaneously painting myself as: a) someone who does not speak English as a first language, b) quite bossy, and c) either excessively compassionate or inexplicably nosy. Meanwhile, my attention shifts back to the flesh-and-blood incarnation of Vomiting Larry and I see him place his now-brimming sick bag clumsily onto the seat next to him and reach for another in the neighbouring pouch. He opens it with only seconds to spare, as another almighty purge gushes from his gaping mouth. It is more than I can bear. I don't wait for an answer, but instead curl my body tightly towards the window and force my head between my knees, sipping the pocket of air between my torso and forehead – desperately trying to convince myself that it has not yet been sullied by his sour cocktail of bile and half-digested food. The steward moves on and my panic is swiftly joined by an unbridled sense of fury. Fury at the steward's neglect to immediately eject Larry from the plane mid-air or to at least make some initial enquiries as to the cause of his demise.

The remainder of the flight, a deeply traumatic hour and forty-five minutes, passes by slowly in an abstract fuzz of snatched breaths, focused observation and panic attacks. Larry is vomiting approximately every fifteen minutes and the only way to cope is to detach completely from my current reality. I am in awe of the people around me, able to read or talk or *eat* in the vicinity of this atrocity, whilst he continues to add to his collection of overflowing paper bags positioned haphazardly on the seat beside him. The scorpions have leapt onto a hamster wheel of obsessive thought, churning together a mass of worst-case scenarios and unanswered questions, turning my mind into a washing machine spin-cycle of undiluted paranoia.

Does he look drunk?

Could it be food poisoning?

Why is he not using the bathroom?

Why are the aeroplane staff ignoring him?

Why aren't they removing his soiled
sick bags from the seat?

Can they really believe it might be motion
sickness, considering the regularity and
intensity of each episode?

If I can smell the vomit, does that mean it has
already entered my system and infected me?

Did he touch any of the same things that I
touched on this plane, allowing the virus
to pass from hand to hand?

Did he know he was sick before he boarded the flight?

How could he be so selfish?

How many days will pass before I definitely
know I have avoided contagion?

How soon could I start to feel sick?

Do I feel sick now?

As the plane finally touches down, Larry seems to have
paused his offensive and I see a stewardess approach his
seat with a casual look of disdain.

'Sir, do you think perhaps you should go and clean
yourself up? The bathroom is free.'

Larry grunts an unintelligible reply but doesn't move
towards the toilet. Instead, he gathers his vomit collection

(I count four bags) as we taxi to a stop, gets up a little unsteadily, and exits the plane as if nothing out of the ordinary has just happened. I remain glued to my seat, protective woollen headpiece still firmly in place, and type out a hysterical message to my mother. These messages are not uncommon after I have experienced a first-hand encounter with a vomiting individual, and they usually follow a similar pattern, in which I rapidly regress to being a seven-year-old child and my mother consequently treats me as such, consoling me with reassurances that are anything but medically founded. A typical exchange might read as follows:

> Oh my god Mum, there was a man throwing up on my flight every fifteen minutes. I was sat reallyclose – I'm so worried I am going to catch it!!! Help!

What?!! Oh no, horrible!
No, you won't catch it, you
have got a strong stomach!
Maybe he was just travel sick?

> There's no way it was travel sickness, it was too intense. It must be contagious. I'll definitely catch it, breathing the same air for two hours!

I'm sure you won't. He could
have been drunk, or had food
poisoning. Even if it was
contagious then it doesn't
mean you will get it.

The messages will continue in this way intermittently for an average of two days, at the end of which I can safely say that forty-eight hours have passed and it can be assumed that I have not caught the virus. (My mother is used to this kind of chaotic correspondence style by this point. She received a similarly frantic phone call whilst I was a student in London, when I, quite urgently, had to seek her advice after having been on the bus sitting beside a woman who'd vomited. I had been minding my own business watching the rain through the steamed-up windows on a bus so packed that people were standing in the aisles and were pressed tightly against the doors, when the woman to my right rummaged through her backpack, pulled out a rectangular lunch box and vomited into it, quite calmly, twice. Pinned to the window seat, I held my breath, hysterically slammed the button to open the doors of the bus, and virtually climbed over the mass of irritated, sweaty bodies like a hungry zombie in order to get to the safety of fresh air and soggy pavement. The position of Lead Reassurer naturally gets passed along from mother to partner as the years go by. Mothers, however, are by definition more suited to the role.)

As the plane's passengers are released, I gather my things, trying to touch as little surface area as possible and steam past the line of stewards, allowing myself a long, deep gulp of air only once I am clear of the tunnel walkway and out in the open space of border control. I unravel the scarf from my head and my sense of reality begins to slot back into place, my cheeks hot from a lack of fresh air and from embarrassment. My eyes find a large digital clock beneath the arrivals board and I make a mental note of the time: forty-eight hours and counting.

Emetophobia is a fear of vomiting or of seeing others being sick. I first heard the word when I was twenty years old and was both relieved and shocked to learn that not only was I amongst other people in the world suffering from this phobia, but also that it was a 'legitimised' fear. No one *likes* to vomit. But for a small proportion of people (an estimated 0.1 per cent of the population, women being four times more likely to suffer than men) the terror associated with catching a virus that might cause you to vomit can begin to influence the way in which you think and how you go about living your life. Travelling in enclosed spaces is an obvious trigger (I'd rather come on my period in a pair of white trousers live on national television than go on the floating Petri dish of a holiday that is a cruise), but there are many other seemingly everyday experiences, objects or locations that can fuel the fire of constant anxiety that rages inside the mind of an emetophobe. Having to shake hands on meeting new people. Using unfamiliar toilets. Visiting hospitals or doctors' surgeries. Attending children's parties. Door handles. Sharing drinks. Supermarket self-check-outs. Undercooked food. Card-machine keypads.

Each presents a new challenge with a familiar goal. How can I navigate the situation before me without anyone suspecting me of being unhinged or thinking of me as rude?

Problem: SHAKING HANDS
Solution: Always ensure both hands are 'accidentally' full or eradicate any need for the shake by pre-empting a greeting with an enthusiastic close-range wave.

Problem: UNFAMILIAR TOILETS
Solution: Touch all handles, taps and surfaces only with a hand covered by an item of clothing (a sleeve/a scarf/the hem of a dress). If possible, send a friend in first and ask for a review.

Problem: HOSPITALS/ DOCTORS' SURGERIES
Solution: Arrive half a minute before the appointment time to reduce contaminated airtime, and sit as far as possible from other people. Do not use bathrooms as they are guaranteed to have been used by other people who are sick in a variety of different ways, otherwise they would not be at the hospital/doctor …

Problem: CHILDREN'S PARTIES
Solution: Avoid entirely unless the party is celebrating your own child. Don't risk the finger buffet.

Problem: DOOR HANDLES
Solution: (See *Unfamiliar Toilets*)

Problem: SHARING DRINKS
Solution: Not under any circumstances. Long-term partner excepted based upon ongoing health observation.

Problem: SUPERMARKET SELF-CHECKOUTS
Solution: Assess health of the checkout operator: if healthy, go to them instead; if peaky, press options onscreen with least-used knuckle (e.g. fourth finger, right hand) never fingertip.

Problem: UNDERCOOKED FOOD
Solution: Evaluate skill level of the chef and decide based upon food type. Not raw egg.

Problem: CARD MACHINE KEYPADS
Solution: Contactless, always, *or* least-used knuckle, in the event of failure.

This is not a healthy list of behaviours, or an example of functioning coping mechanisms, but simply the reality of some of the ways in which I have adapted my everyday life to avoid contagion. One of the most effective strategies to tackle sickness prevention and a common hallmark of obsessive-compulsive behaviour is excessive hand-washing – with which I have had a lifelong and passionate love affair. Due to the generally positive and beneficial associations with hand-washing, it is not a compulsion I have to hide, or rather the extent of it is rarely witnessed by other people, as it mostly takes place in the privacy of my home or a public bathroom. I used to consider hand cream an unnecessary luxury. A last-resort Christmas gift for distant great-aunts or well-meaning grandmas. But it has now become an essential part of my daily routine, in order to remain in possession of two skin-covered hands by the time I reach old age.

In my early twenties, there was a point at which the hand-washing and my panic attacks, driven by a blanket anxiety I couldn't temper, began to overwhelm me. I was referred by my doctor for a course of cognitive behavioural therapy (CBT), often the first port of call for OCD treatment. I did a fair amount of research about this type of therapy and, somewhere along the way, I read that 'exposure therapy' can be an element of the CBT plan, and consequently that one small element became my total obsession. As you can imagine, the sessions did not go as planned. I arrived at my first session utterly convinced that before the course was finished I would be forced to place both hands on the inside of a toilet bowl and made to lick them clean in order to expose myself to a level of bacteria so high that

I would become violently sick and in turn address my fear of vomiting. In my mind, when treating OCD in relation to emetophobia I could not imagine what else exposure therapy might be if not French kissing norovirus patients, touching toilet seats and not washing your hands for an entire year ... None of which subsequently happened to me, of course, due to the fact that, firstly, exposure therapy was never even mentioned in our sessions, and, secondly, because I did everything in my power to convince my therapist from day one that I was recovering at a rate of knots.

Some years later I came across an article in a magazine about a man who was suffering from a brain tumour. Through some complication concerning the intracranial process, he experienced 'spontaneous vomiting' as a primary symptom, whereby his tumour was causing direct stimulation of the vomiting centre in his brain, and as a result he was throwing up without any warning or any prior preparatory nausea. I remembered this curious symptom, because although the circumstances of his illness were utterly harrowing, this standalone symptom itself struck me as the optimal way in which to experience vomiting, should it be *absolutely* necessary for survival in moments of infection or self-protection. It felt primal somehow. Like a cat who has eaten too much and throws up nonchalantly onto the grass, before going about the rest of its day without so much as a second thought about what just occurred. No agonising pacing before the bathroom door waiting for endless nausea to give way to its inevitable purge. No dreadful slow kneel to position yourself over the toilet bowl as the bile rises in your throat and you prepare to take aim. The months of unresolved nausea I experienced as a child had rendered me incapable of coping with this necessary biological preparation. I can count on one finger the times I have physically vomited as an adult (twenty-four years old, a twelve-hour virus, vomited once after a day of nausea whilst my then-boyfriend ate a takeaway curry on the sofa next to me), my will against it has become so strong. And so, I adapt. And avoid. And I wash my hands.

Looking down at them now, veiny, long-fingered and beginning to show the first signs of age in the spidery wrinkles crawling across my knuckles, I can see the legacy of my secret rituals nestled in the shallow webbing between each digit. A map of parched dermis, small patches of skin peeling and cracking to form a fragmented interconnected armour, comforting in its familiarity. I stretch my fingers wide and the skin pulls taut over my palm as if the fit is just a little too tight. The brittle fold between thumb and forefinger is paper dry, and I can't help but manipulate those creases, pushing the limits of elasticity, as a delicate fissure forms in front of me, releasing a hairline tributary of blood that disappears almost immediately into the thirsty plain beneath. I reach for a tube of grandma's finest and allow the life to return slowly to my skin, smoothing the cool cream over and over again into the cracks – a kind of reverse hand-washing – until I am satisfied, once again, that this skin belongs to me.

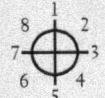

GAS COOKER RITUAL

☒ Stand facing the cooker.

☒ Observe the four hob buttons for any sign of misalignment.

☒ Touch each button with your right hand, whilst saying the number of the button aloud:

☒ Move from left to right:

1, 2, 3, 4.

☒ Repeat backwards from right to left:

4, 3, 2, 1.

☒ Now repeat the action from left to right, but this time count from 1 to 8 on each button before moving to the next.

☒ Repeat backwards from right to left.

☒ As the whole ritual began moving left to right, then it is unfair on the right-hand side, so begin the same ritual as above, but starting this time from right to left.

☒ First count, 2, 3, 4 on each button, then repeat with a prolonged count of 1 to 8 on each.

☒ Move on when fully satisfied.

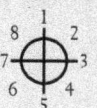

☒ Next is a sensory check.

☒ Bend down so the underside of the hob is at eye level.

☒ Visually check for signs of a blue flame, accompanied by mental count of 1 to 8 whilst looking at each burner. Do this for all four burners, four times, each time starting on a different burner so the check is fair.

☒ Inhale slowly to check for the smell of gas.

☒ Return to standing, then perform a visual check for identical alignment of all four buttons, whilst counting 1 to 8 at rapid speed.

☒ If still unsatisfied after repeating the ritual, take four photographs of the cooker from different angles for visual reassurance later in the day.

Chapter Four

HOMING

*'Scorpions might use their pectines to acquire
and store matrices of chemical and textural
information during homebound journeys and
use these memories to retrace paths...'*

Douglas D. Gaffin & Brad P. Brayfield, 'Exploring the chemo-textural
familiarity hypothesis for scorpion navigation', *BioOne*

Choose your own OCD adventure!

HOME

You wake up, head throbbing after a night full of bad dreams. Nightmares of death and destruction. You have a sour taste in your mouth, so you drink a glass of water to wash away this most unfavourable start to your day. The sunshine streams through the gap in your curtains, reminding you of the many possible adventures that lie ahead. It takes you longer than usual to get dressed – after all, you have a busy day in front of you and you want to look your best. It's not every day that you attend a party *and* leave to go on holiday … You'd better get going, or you'll never make it in time!

Every minute counts as you quickly pack your rucksack, locate your passport and race downstairs. You have many rituals to complete before you leave the house: you haven't yet checked the cooker, the light switches or the taps. Do you waste precious minutes by completing your checks or do you leave the house now and do them next time?

Complete checks:
go to box ONE

Leave the house:
go to box EIGHT

ONE

You haven't lost too much time, but you have gained a sense of achievement and security. As you close the front door behind you, rucksack in hand, you are pleased to hear no running water, are elated to see the lights turned off and the curtains drawn, and there is not a whiff of gas in the air. Well done, you! You are distracted by the sound of your phone ringing in your pocket as the door clicks shut, and you realise, to your horror – you have left your house keys on the kitchen table! You cancel the call, irritated, and think about your next move. Should you accept the door is closed and skip double-locking it? Or search frantically through your many phone notes to try and find the lockbox code and retrieve your spare key?

Accept the door is closed:
go to box TEN

Retrieve the key and lock the door:
go to box TWO

TWO

Door now safely locked, you can check to see who was calling you. It was the friend whose birthday party you are attending, before you have to catch a flight to the holiday destination of your dreams later today. They tell you that all public transport in the area is down – just your luck! You wait ten minutes for a taxi, but lose patience as you know that the party has already begun. Nearby you spot a rental bike leaning against a wall and check the app to see if it is available. As you tip the bike to scan the code, a small amount of water escapes the frame and covers the handlebars. Strange… you don't remember it raining recently? Unsure of what exactly this liquid could be, you decide that there are really only two choices:

Take the bike to get there faster:
go to box NINE

Choose to walk (what the hell is that liquid?):
go to box THREE

THREE

It is a pleasant walk to your friend's house, if a little long, but you are thankful for the sun on your back and the late-summer breeze caressing your skin. You count the steps as your feet hit the ground, beating out a comforting rhythm, and drop your eyes to notice the way your left foot turns in slightly when you walk. As you try to correct it, you spot a large pothole in the road up ahead. You are mesmerised by the symmetry of this hole and imagine how nice it would feel to place your feet either side of it and count each of its soft, curved corners until you could move on to the next corner and start again. Each time a count of 8. But there are people approaching from the other direction, and you could risk looking stupid or mad … Do you:

Ignore the pothole and keep walking:
go to box TEN

Count the corners and risk damaging
your perceived sanity:
go to box FOUR

FOUR

You arrive at the party a little tired and sweaty, but no one seems to mind as you are invited into a room full of friendly faces, good music and lots of cake! Time seems to run away from you, as you are deep in conversation with your best friend and barely even notice the light begin to change as late morning becomes late afternoon, and you check your watch after what feels like five minutes to see that it is soon time to leave for the airport. Someone hands you a slice of chocolate cake, which you scoff greedily, and you wish everyone a hasty goodbye as you rush towards the exit, a drunken rendition of 'Happy Birthday' floating down from the top floor. As you get to the hallway of the apartment building, you remember you have forgotten to wash your hands before leaving. It is three flights of stairs back up to your friend's apartment, where you could use her bathroom to clean up – after all, you *did* shake a lot of hands …

Don't clean up; leave for the airport:
go to box TWELVE

Climb the stairs and wash your hands:
go to box FIVE

FIVE

This time you're in luck! A taxi pulls up to the kerb and drops a passenger just across the road from you, so you take the opportunity to jump in and make your way to the airport with plenty of time to spare. You watch the world fly by your window in a blur and rest your head against the glass, conserving your energy for the flight you are about to catch. Your eyes fall to your lap and you let out a groan as you notice a dirty smear on your new trousers. How did that get there? It could be chocolate cake, carelessly dropped during your hasty retreat. Perhaps it is dirt, or even *faeces*, picked up whilst brushing against the rental bike earlier, or sharing the toilet at your friend's party with such a large group of people... You consider your options:

Taste the smear to see if it's chocolate:
go to box TWELVE

Steer clear of the smear and change
clothes at the airport:
go to box SIX

Touch the smear to identify its texture:
go to box NINE

SIX

You emerge from the airport toilets in a fresh set of clothes, ready for your next adventure – thank goodness you packed several outfits for your holiday! You look around the airport, enjoying the buzz of excitement in the air, so many people jetting off to pastures new. Resisting duty-free, you take a seat at a cafe next to your gate and order yourself a little treat. As you finally start to relax and allow images of sandy beaches and clear blue skies to flood your head, an announcement rings out over the speakers, disturbing your perfect daydream.

'Apologies, but flight ****** to ****** has been delayed. Please check the board for further information.'

Delayed! There was no warning about this online, no air-traffic control incidents, no bad weather. It must be a technical fault, you think. You heart rate climbs dramatically, your thoughts beginning to spiral. You're uncertain of whether you are being silly or whether there really could be something wrong with the plane. What do you do?

Take your chances and get on the plane:
go to box SEVEN

Something's not right: don't board the plane:
go to box ELEVEN

SEVEN

Any dark thoughts you had about boarding the plane are immediately banished when you arrive at your row only to be told there is a free upgrade on offer if you would like to take it. Naturally, you jump at the chance and soon you are settling in to your spacious new seat, your eyelids growing heavy with fatigue. It has been a long day, and it is only when the sound of the engines thundering signal the oncoming departure that you realise you haven't followed your usual routine. It has always been customary to carry a packet of Werther's Originals with you on every flight to consume upon take-off and landing. You have always been loyal to this tradition, for fear of something awful happening should you forget. But you are stuck in the window seat and your luggage is in the compartment above. With only seconds until you reach the runway, do you leave your seat, squeeze past your neighbour and fetch your sweets from the locker overhead, or do you leave them be and surrender to the temptation of sleep?

Fetch the sweets:
go to box ELEVEN

Surrender to sleep:
go to box THIRTEEN

EIGHT

You have left the gas on! The candle that you failed to check has ignited the gas in the air and burned down your house, everything you own has been reduced to ashes. Go back **HOME** to sob in the rubble and beg your insurance company for money.

NINE

You have been poisoned by a powerful nerve agent! You die a short and extremely painful death, before your body is returned back **HOME** ahead of a post-mortem and a full investigation.

TEN

All of your family and friends spontaneously come down with a mysterious illness and die. Return **HOME** to organise the funerals.

ELEVEN

You continue to live a relatively happy and successful life, free of calamitous air-travel incidents, but due to increased life expectancy and the unavoidable presence of micro-plastics in virtually everything around us, you inevitably contract a life-threatening disease. Return **HOME** to say your goodbyes.

TWELVE

You contract a vomiting bug. Go **HOME** to make a full, but very slow and agonising, recovery.

THIRTEEN

The plane hits a violent thunderstorm mid-flight and spirals out of control, crashing into a remote rainforest. There are no survivors. What remains of your body, along with your belongings and an untouched packet of Werther's Originals, are returned to your **HOME**.

**PLAY AGAIN AND SEE WHERE
THE ADVENTURE TAKES YOU!**

Chapter Five

NOCTURNE

'This species is a strictly nocturnal sit-and-wait
predator. Individuals spend only a small proportion of
apparently suitable nights foraging on the surface;
the remainder are spent in a deep burrow.'

Richard Bradley, 'The Influence of Weather and Biotic Factors
on the Behaviour of the Scorpion (Paruroctonus utahensis)'

2021. A MONDAY. 1.30AM

I am awoken by a cacophony of voices in the street outside my house. The neighbours are congregating with some friends beneath my bedroom window, exchanging inebriated farewells at the same maddening volume favoured by sports teachers and town criers. The climactic trill of a pop song can be heard streaming from the window of an idling taxi as the guests pile clumsily inside. The metal frame of my bed shudders slightly when the car door slams shut, carrying the muffled sound of laughter off into the night. I close my eyes and listen to the seeds of yet another argument being planted next door, as the hosts discard their united front, worn fleetingly and for company's sake, before making their leaden retreat back inside to yell through the paper-thin walls that separate our homes.

The air in my room is torrid and it clings to my skin like the dry, close heat of a desert. I roll onto my back, pleading silently for sleep to come, but I already know that I am no longer alone here in the dark. Within moments I can hear the scurry of tiny legs reverberating in my skull, the familiar *clack-clack* of armoured bodies. Glistening, black forms dart back and forth across my vision and a tingling sensation shoots down my spine. I sit up, scanning my body for the smallest movement, when I feel a short, sharp sting inside my chest. *Not again.*

My breath quickens as a white-hot pressure starts to build beneath my heart. The sensation of burning. Curling myself inwards, I wrap my arms tight around my knees in a desperate attempt to crush my twitching assailants before they launch another senseless attack.

My defences crumble for just a moment, but a moment is all they need and the scorpions act quickly, stirring panic into my blood as a terrible thought strikes me.

The butter lettuce.

'Would you like any sides with that?' chirps our waitress, looking at me with big blinking eyes. It is the end of summer and alongside the many other customers seated on this terrace, my partner and I are desperately upholding the delusion that it is still warm enough to eat outside without a jacket.

'Umm.' I throw a look to him across the table; I know he thinks we've ordered enough already. 'What's good here? What would you recommend?'

'Well, I usually go for the sweet potato fries, but I've heard the butter lettuce is really nice ...' She trails off, her eyebrows rising in unison with her shoulders, a move designed to let us know that she won't be judging us either way.

I bite my lip in mock contemplation, already certain that I want the fries. I feel her eyes on me as I examine the menu I've been holding for the last fifteen minutes. 'Does it come with anything?'

A frown dances across her face. 'No, it's just, sort of … lettuce. With a dressing on it.'

'Oh, right, great!' I say, in a voice higher and more enthusiastic than I had intended. 'We'll have the butter lettuce then please.' I gather up the menus without a second thought and bundle them into her hands, confident I have made the right decision. A decision so achingly chic, I immediately order a glass of champagne to complement it. I don't even like champagne.

Sometime later, drunk on peanuts and social contact, I barely notice when the food finally arrives at our table. The waitress distributes each dish with a flourish, but saves the salad until last, placing it proudly next to my plate.

I take a moment to consider it, this beautiful bouquet of green. It is a wholesome creation, practically experimental in its simplicity. There's an unmistakeable arrogance to it, touched by the kind of unassuming genius that lands you a Michelin star and a judging spot on *MasterChef*. A butter lettuce, in its entirety, sawn roughly in half (almost certainly unwashed) and served with one delicate splash of French mustard vinaigrette.

But as our waitress is summoned to the neighbouring table, I begin to inspect it more closely, and my stomach drops. I spot it instantly. A small cluster of brown spots gathered along the rim of one of the leaves several layers down, tucked out of sight. Tiny uneven circles of rot like miniature cigarette burns. As if the Borrowers had smoked cigars in the salad drawer and stubbed their smouldering butts out on the surface of the lettuce. But it is only one leaf, and I count just four spots. Four. A friendly number, all things considered. I like fours. I deal very frequently with fours.

The edges curl gently towards me, tinged with half an inch of muddy brown. I'm two glasses of champagne deep and it's clear I've become giddy with careless abandon. I step momentarily out of my body and watch myself with something close to awe as I slice off a large chunk of the lettuce, brown spots and all and stuff it greedily into my mouth, not even stopping to check the leaves beneath. I am several chews in when I crunch something hard. I know exactly what it is. I convince myself it is a rogue piece of black peppercorn, the tough organic shell splitting open between my teeth. But I know deep down that my cavalier attitude has cost me dearly, and I have hit upon some grit secreted amongst the folds of green. Something shifts imperceptibly inside my head and I have the sense that hundreds of tiny pairs of eyes are watching me from within, pincers poised and ready to take hold. I challenge the fear beginning to flood my body. All I want to do is spit it out. To deposit this masticated mess inside the white linen napkin that is draped delicately across my knees. To dig my fingers deep inside my cheeks and extract the offending piece of dirt, stripping my mouth clean of potential infection. But I am not in the privacy of my own home, neither am I a child rejecting an unfamiliar vegetable, and – for whatever reason – I am feeling brave tonight, so (desperate to be a normal person for just one evening of my life) I try my best to forget about it. I force myself to swallow and it slides uneventfully down my throat. An occurrence so lacking in the peril and significance I have bestowed upon it, that I feel triumphant when nothing happens. The mouth across from me is moving in slow motion and gradually I tune back in to the conversation. Something about a book adaptation – German colonialism in Africa? Agreeing a little too loudly, I take in my surroundings with a fresh sense of wonder. The world around me completely unaware that I have just taken the first courageous steps towards a life free from obsession. I have drawn my sword against the scorpions; and this time, I refused to back away. I take a deep breath, a sip of water, and dive headlong into my new-found heroism.

Several hours later, I am lying in bed facing my imminent death, with only myself to blame. *How could I have been so stupid?* I begin to bargain with … who? Myself? The universe?

If I [future selfless act*] then spare me the [possible consequences of my actions**] now. I promise I won't do it again.

The panic grows inside me and I consider my options. Call an ambulance? The Food Standards Agency? My mother? The searing pain in my heart is growing and my body starts to writhe and twist in an attempt to stave off the inevitable. I scroll through my mental archives searching the limited section on science. Is there anything that I have learned in my thirty-four years on this planet that could support my newly minted theory that there may in fact be a type of bacteria found in butter lettuce that, if it makes its way into the body and is absorbed into the blood, can actually stop the heart dead? I realise with terrifying certainty that ... I don't know. I search the outer reaches of my mind for some definitive evidence to the contrary, but all I see is the squirming horde scurrying to block my way.

And so it must be. The end of my journey on Earth could fast be approaching, and I look at the clock to watch my final hours – or perhaps even minutes – tick by in passive horror. It appears I have already devoted two hours to in-depth situational analysis and am disturbed to discover that I am none the wiser.

It's 3.53am. I hate 3s.

---

* *Volunteer/donate to charity/stop ignoring calls from friends.*
** *Food poisoning/cardiac arrest/parasites.*

No! I curse myself for making my second fatal mistake of the evening. Offending the number 3. I am sure to receive a particularly merciless kind of karma for that thought. A payback that awaits me the next time I stand next to someone with a contagious illness, or board a plane, or need a loved one to recover from a serious operation. I will see that number 3 somewhere in a row of seats, a smattering of stones on a pavement, or scrawled innocently across a jumper – and it will spell out my impending doom. An odd number (not a good start) that has most definitely been offended by my negative thought-crime against it and will come back to teach me a lesson. I am certain of it. I hold my hand flat against my heart to check it is still beating, something I do most nights as I am falling asleep. I wait for eight life-sustaining thumps to pass before I remove my hand, then repeat the action, just to be sure. My heart is definitely still beating – but I think it might be going too fast. Much, much too fast, and increasing by the minute. I feel a prickle of sweat under my arms, like a network of tiny dams all bursting their banks simultaneously, coating my body with a damp sheen. I stare into the darkness hoping to pluck some reassuring titbit of information from the depths of my brain.

Before the days of Apple Macs and browser history, I consulted a book called *Back to Eden* by Jethro Kloss. It is still one of the thickest books I own, and it provided the essential service of collating and alphabetising all the major illnesses that the human body could possibly suffer from. I have memorised the symptoms of most major diseases, and in any one evening I can have developed a particularly aggressive and very rare type of cancer, a fast-moving blood clot hellbent on travelling to my brain, or sometimes even a collapsed lung or two. Conveniently for me, technology has moved on, and I have a whole new world of categorised symptoms at my fingertips. Diseases I didn't even know existed. And so it transpires that the middle of the night is my chance to spend some quality time with Dr Google.

Dr Google is never judgemental, is always impeccably well informed, and deals only with cold, hard facts. If you feel *this*, then you may have *that*. Speedy, ambitious diagnoses at the click of a button. (With the gifts of hindsight and daylight I am able to rationalise that it is highly likely that the doctor is in cahoots with the scorpions, but a brain stuck in the tumultuous storm of obsessive thought is a difficult one to reason with). I begin my consultation.

butter lettuce heart attack, butter lettuce bacteria, heart parasite lettuce, rare death butter lettuce heart, poison lettuce, woman dies butter lettuce, heart attack signs, how to slow down heartbeat, how do I know if my heart is beating too fast, water on the heart, heart attack water

Water. I should drink some water. That will help. I scramble around in the darkness, my hand rhythmically patting the space beside my bed until I find what I am looking for. As I bring the glass to my lips, I feel a sudden pressure surge inside my skull. The restless swarm of creatures jostling to push a new idea to the forefront of my mind. They are well practised and succeed within seconds. Powerless, I feel the thought click firmly into place.

What if someone entered my room when I was asleep and replaced the water in my glass with oil?

These giant leaps of fancy somehow only seem plausible in the dead of night, yet at the same time, they make total, uncomplicated sense. From somewhere in the darkness, I remember that I read just days ago that the substance I use to fill my (wildly impractical) bedside oil lamps can easily kill a child, and, if ingested, can cause irreparable damage to a pair of adult lungs. It is at times like this that I question my attraction to the Victorian gloom aesthetic that inspired me to buy a pair of lamps that require regular refilling with a potentially hazardous liquid. My mouth is so dry. Maybe the water will flush out the bacteria from the butter lettuce, in which case it is essential that I take a sip, but how can I be absolutely sure that I am not drinking oil? The palpitations that have been hopping and skipping in my chest begin to pick up speed and I know I mustn't delay any longer. I throw my head back taking several big gulps of the unclassified liquid, allowing it momentarily to cool the fire in my heart. It isn't long before I am back with the doctor.

lamp oil smell, can oil be odourless, what does
oil taste like, drinking lamp oil, permanent lung
damage oil, oil in lungs breathless, lamp oil
ingestion death

Death preoccupies most humans from time to time, but
for me it is not just a slow ticking clock to be ignored until
I am old and frail, or an occasional fleeting awareness of
my mortality when a distant relative dies, but a constant,
looming presence that stokes my fear daily and has stolen
countless hours of my sleeping life. Insomnia has been my
loyal bedfellow for almost two decades. My parents were
always late to bed and early risers, so sleep never seemed
important when I was small. There was always too much
to think about, too much to do. After many years of practice, I can survive on very little sleep a night, and so instead
I reserve my moonlit hours for high-octane worrying.

There is a special kind of mysticism that takes hold of
me at night, those hours that feel lost to reality, existing in
another realm. The real world of daylight and truth gives
way to a never-ending stretch of time in which everything
feels closer, heavier, yet totally unreachable. My mind
has always been most active after dark. I am continually inspired and seduced by its potential for beauty and
creativity, but as long as I am awake and my mind is open,
then my scorpions have all the space and time they need
to turn this sense of magic into melancholy and danger.
These creatures are always battling for the spotlight, for

my undivided attention, and it is the night that gifts it to them in a most generous and concentrated way. I believe it was Freud who made the link between a child's resistance to falling asleep and a fear of dying, whether or not this was a conscious connection on the child's part. He determined that sleep represented what I think of as a kind of mini-death, an unknown black hole into which we are supposed to willingly succumb without a fight, and without conclusive evidence as to where exactly we are going, or if we will ever return. It is no coincidence, then, that a brain susceptible to a disorder such as OCD – devoid of logic and drawn in by the most mundane of fantasies – might become locked in to a pattern of thought that begins with a relatively harmless rumination and inevitably circles back to an all-consuming obsession with one's own mortality. A life knitted together by a series of narrowly avoided mini-deaths.

A relatively recent addition to my personal disaster scenario back-catalogue is the notion that every time I go to receive a vaccine or a blood test at the doctors, I am convinced the nurse is going to accidentally inject a bubble of air into my veins that will travel to my brain or heart causing a fatal stroke or heart attack. I understand that this sort of occurrence is extremely unlikely – in fact I have never heard of it having happened to someone, only that it *could* be possible – and so, naturally, I researched the outcome of that rare possibility (spoiler: it's death). Having then tried to determine if modern syringes are designed to eliminate these air bubbles from ever occurring, I couldn't find definitive evidence that reassured me that every syringe was built to be death-proof, therefore leaving me to rely entirely upon the frighteningly analogue testing method I have observed of 'flicking the syringe' with one's middle finger several times. I have no doubt that a nurse or a doctor will read the above with a generous dose of eye-rolling, irritated at my ignorance to what must seem such an obviously simple determination, but in my distorted mind the margin for human error feels just a little bit too large. In these instances, my strong inclination to want to be protected against any number of illnesses a vaccine can prevent, or to rapidly receive results of a blood test to ensure I don't have any hidden diseases, just about overrides my fear of the air bubble. So instead of refusing the injection, I merely think about it for hours afterwards, mentally scanning different parts of my body for rogue intravenous air pockets. Is my arm aching? Do I have a headache? Is that a pain in my chest? Ruminations like these can cover anything from butter lettuce to bathroom taps, but they almost always end with death.

And that is how it ends tonight, with the inevitable deal being struck. I gather myself, heart racing, and take a long deep breath as I summon the scorpions. They are restless, and I know I have to move quickly. I must hold on to the flicker of rational thought visible through this thrumming hive of activity. I implore:

Please don't let death take me now. I will be better, I won't take risks with my health, I won't take my beating heart for granted. Delay my demise and I will put something good into this world. I will take care of you. I will perform my routines every day, without fail, for longer. I will invent new ones. Show you how devoted I am. I will listen when you call on me. I will trust you to keep me safe. Give me one more chance and I will prove myself. I just need time. Not tonight, I am not ready to go. Calm this pounding in my chest – I can't catch my breath. Please. It hurts. It is going too fast. It shouldn't be this fast. Make it stop. Make it stop. Make it stop.

I open my eyes, both hands covering my heart, and realise the room has descended into anechoic silence. They have accepted the deal. I look over to my partner, the sleeping figure beside me, my head lighter in defeat, and he turns to settle into a new position, enjoying a slumber so deep that my stomach twists with envy. I shuffle slowly backwards, tucking my feet between the warm crook of his knees. And as the dawn light breaks through a gap in the curtains and my body finally surrenders to sleep, a lone thought remains, knocking softly against the walls of my cranium like a lullaby.

Should have had the fries.

Should have had the fries.

Should have had the fries.

Ballad of the Scorpion Lady

There once was a woman whose head
Gave birth to a scorpion bed.
But try as she might,
They wouldn't take flight,
So she counted some corners instead.

Chapter Six

SUBTERFUGE

subterfuge (/ˈsʌbtəfjuː(d)ʒ/) – *deceit used in order to achieve one's goal.*

Psssst. Psssssssssssssst.

What?

Are you awake?

No.

What are you doing?

. . .

What are you doing?

Nothing.

Were you sleeping?

I was trying.

Are you tired?

Yes.

Does your body feel tired?

Yes. Move over, I can feel your claws.

Maybe you're sick.

I don't feel sick. I'm just tired.

Are you sure?

. . .

Are you sure you don't feel sick?

I don't think so.

Cancer makes you feel tired.

Cancer? What kind of cancer.

Every kind.

I don't have cancer.

How do you know?

I don't have any symptoms.

The worst ones don't have any symptoms.

Until the end.

I need to sleep.

You could catch it early. If you act now.

It's 4am.

Never too late to check.

Oh God, I just heard.

Heard what?

You have cancer.

I don't have cancer.

Who has cancer?

Nobody.

Well, that's not true, is it.

It's actually very common.

She could have cancer.

She could have cancer.

You could have cancer.

Why would I have cancer?!

It's very common.

Very common. 1 in 2.

1 in 2 ... She won't like those odds.

... I don't like those odds.

Are you sure you don't feel sick?

Does your stomach feel OK?

Well, now you mention it ...

I knew you felt sick, I could sense it.

Wake the others.

No, don't wake the others. I'm fine.

You're sick.

We should wake the others.

Just in case.

Just in case.

Do you think you might vomit?

Do YOU think I might vomit?

It is possible. I mean, if you feel sick …

Oh God, she's going to vomit.

But I don't think I do feel sick.

Why is your stomach churning then?

I can hear it from here!

I think I'm nervous. You're making me nervous.

You can't get sick from nerves.

You must have a bug.

What do you mean I could catch it early if I 'act now'?

Maybe you should call someone.

Who?

When was the last time you had a scan?

Your mother.

I'm not calling my mother. She'll be asleep.

Just message her then.

Just message her.

…

OK. A quick message.

Are you up? I feel sick, I'm worried I might be sick. I won't be sick, will I? I haven't been around anyone who has been ill. I haven't eaten anything bad …
Even if I HAD been near to someone ill, then that doesn't mean I would catch it, does it? X

Good, that's very good.

I can't remember …

Can't remember what?

When I last had a scan.

It was a very long time ago.

Very long.

Long enough for something to grow.

You wouldn't even know about it.

It's sneaky like that.

Interesting, that you … can't remember.

Why is that interesting?

Well, didn't you have pins and needles quite recently?

What's that got to do with anything?

The others are here.

Move over, I can feel your claws!

It just seems neurological, that's all.

Tell them to go. I can't think.

Definitely neurological. It's all linked.

I. Can't. Think.

Must be neurological

Shut up!

Calm down.

Try to stay calm. We're all here.

I AM CALM!!!

Oh no! When did it come on?
I'm sure you'll be fine darling.
Wish I could help. Is there
anyone there with you? Xxxxx

We're all here. Tell her we're here.

No, don't tell her.

She doesn't like us.

She thinks we mislead you.

Tell her we're here.

I don't want you here! This is your fault!

Do you want to be alone?

We can leave you alone, if that's what you want.

To be sick on your own.

I don't want to be sick. Please don't leave—

But you said you didn't need us?

You said you didn't want us—

Don't leave.

Well.

You've upset us now.

I didn't mean to.

But you have.

You've pushed your luck.

You ARE very lucky not to have been sick for so long.

Not to have broken a bone.

You should be careful, with luck like that.

It always runs out.

Always.

Something bad could happen ...

Like what?

... taking things for granted like that.

LIKE WHAT???????

...

...

...

Sorry I shouted. Like what?

Death.

Death!

Most probably.

Who?

Who do you love the most?

That's not fair.

Aren't you lucky?

So lucky.

Isn't she lucky!

Am I lucky?

I guess I could be lucky.

You want to hold on to luck like that.

Yes, I do. But how?

We could help.

You could?

Absolutely.

It would be our pleasure.

All of our pleasure.

I feel very hot. Is it hot in here?

You could have a fever.

We're all here. It's crowded.

It is hot. We're all here.

HOW could you help??

Maybe you should call a doctor.

You must try to stay calm.

I think I feel sick.

Go and stand by the toilet.

There are too many of you.

Go and stand by the toilet.

I don't want to.

You have to! It's happening!

Please ... I'll do anything ...

Wouldn't it be sad for that luck to run out.

You had a good run.

I'm going to stand by the toilet!

Just calm down.

You're not well.

What's that sound???

Nothing. It's just us.

No one else is here.

Stop talking all at once.

I can't hear anything—

You seem a bit paranoid.

Try counting, that might help.

Eight deep breaths.

Eight deep breaths.

Doctors aren't open at this time of night, are they?

In and out.

In and out.

Call 111.

If you dig your thumbnails into the tips of your
middle finger on each hand you won't throw up.

What? Why?

Trust me.

Trust us.

Do it eight times.

That makes no sense.

Trust us. We can help you.

I think I should call the emergency doctor.

My chest feels tight —

> *All you have to do is count.*

> *It's so simple. We'll do the rest.*

Do you promise I won't get sick?

> *We promise.*

You'll stay with me?

> *Of course we will.*

> *Of course we will.*

Are you ok?
Have you been sick?
Xxxxxx

I'm doing it, I'm digging my nails in.

1, 2, 3, 4, 5, 6, 7, 8.

Hello?

1. 2. 3. 4. 5. 6. 7. 8.

...

...

Hello. Are you there?

...

Has it worked?

I can't feel your claws. Are you there?

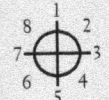

TAP RITUAL

☒ Begin with your hand palm up, hovering beneath the kitchen tap to check for drips.

1, 2, 3, 4, 5, 6, 7, 8.

☒ Turn your hand over, palm facing down.

1, 2, 3, 4, 5, 6, 7, 8.

☒ Repeat the action. This time start with your palm facing down, 1, 2, 3, 4, 5, 6, 7, 8.

☒ Then turn your hand over, palm facing up.

1, 2, 3, 4, 5, 6, 7, 8.

☒ Press your thumb against the handle of the faucet and apply gentle pressure eight times to make sure the tap is closed.

☒ Repeat the entire sequence.

☒ Lean close to the tap to visually confirm that no water is escaping.

☒ Frame the tap with your eyes, so the tap is in the centre of the kitchen tile behind it. Now, with your eyes closed, count: 1, 2, 3, 4, 5, 6, 7, 8.

☒ If you are interrupted, you must begin the ritual again.

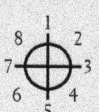

Chapter Seven

HIBERNATION

'The scorpion has the ability to spring quickly to
the hunt when the opportunity presents itself –
a gift that many hibernating species lack.'

National Geographic, nationalgeographic.com

I was shooting a film in Los Angeles during the winter of 2019 when news first began to circulate about a virus wreaking havoc in Wuhan, China. In hindsight I look back on those first few months like much of the rest of the world: as if watching the opening to a zombie apocalypse film. The trickle of abstract news stories expanding to become a daily bombardment of terror. The disassociation and denial giving way to a grave dose of reality on our doorsteps. Inconceivable events changing each of our lives in ways we never could have imagined. I arrived back home only two weeks before the UK was plunged into its first total lockdown. Visiting my family just a few days before travel was banned or bubbles invented, I barely had time to catch my breath before settling into what we now know as one of the most challenging and devastating years in our recent history.

On paper, the ingredients of a global pandemic detail a potentially disastrous recipe for an OCD sufferer such as myself. Extended periods of time spent entirely alone, a killer virus spreading quicker than it could be controlled (and in ways we did not yet understand), and a dramatic and sudden upheaval of our daily routines. For someone who had devoted a large portion of her life to worrying about health, death and infection control, I was surprised, and perhaps even a little ashamed, to find that I was struck almost immediately by an awful sense of calm.

There is a school of thought that suggests people with chronic depressive or anxiety disorders cope better in times of complete crisis. When one dedicates considerable time and energy to cataloguing a glut of worst-case scenarios and formulating action plans for each of these traumatic eventualities, it can come as an unexpected and overwhelming relief when something happens that actually forces one to act upon these absurd game plans. So, as the spread of Covid-19 began to dominate our very existence and infect our sense of normality, a new reality came to fruition – one previously only imaginable in the depths of an overactive mind – and the world finally aligned with my experience of the everyday.

Scorpions can hibernate for long periods of time. Mine have often tricked me into thinking they have moved on entirely until something triggers their return, be that a new environment, a stressful life event, or even just a rogue snowball of a thought. I had expected the Covid-19 pandemic to be one such life event, but whilst the world was gripped by terror and grief, I began to feel safer than ever in my private little bubble. Lockdown for me was spent alone in a two-bedroom flat in North London, with only my little grey cat for company. My partner and I spent most of it apart, due to our being in separate countries at the time, and so I settled into a routine of comforting invariability. Feed cat, feed self, watch the news, google Covid symptoms, take a short walk around the block, 5pm glass of red wine (to numb the horror of the latest death toll), try to read (fail to read), obsessively play the same four songs into the ground (a terrible habit of mine, causing me to periodically detest most of the music I love), then sleep (albeit restlessly). I went days without speaking any words out loud, and my long-held childhood fantasy of developing selective mutism (for which I blame Ariel's alluringly speechless on-land manifestation in *The Little Mermaid*) became a reality. The now-enforced lack of social contact was something I had been trying to engineer in my own life for years. The anxiety of avoiding gatherings, dodging messages and unexpectedly bumping into people I knew (shudder) was eradicated without any influence or effort on my part. When weaving a web of lies to avoid a meeting, a person or an event, it is important to remember that even if said web belongs to the most delicate of money spiders – a distant cousin twice removed from the thick, sticky film of a tarantula's silken burrow – the chances are you will get caught up in it regardless. Stripped of the need to agonise over ways in which to excuse myself, I felt a renewed strength take hold. A calm ease with myself and the space around me permeated into the atmosphere, the furniture; even the cat was more agreeable than ever.

Coupled with this welcome social castration was an order to leave our houses as *little* as possible, for limited pockets of time. Leaving the house has always been, for me, a drawn-out nightmare of an event. A time when my scorpions are at their most productive, doling out orders and demands, questioning my every move. Naturally, leaving the house less frequently meant that my routines became fewer. Not only were they performed less often, but the reduced periods for which we were allowed to 'take the air', like prisoners enjoying yard time, allowed for a smaller window in which catastrophic disasters could occur inside my apartment whilst I was elsewhere. If I had somehow unknowingly laid the foundations for a mistake that would cause any number of things to burst into flames whilst I was gone, then surely only having left the house for a brief fifteen-minute stroll would afford me the chance to salvage the last of my most treasured belongings and put a stop to the raging inferno before it completely obliterated my home? The final and perhaps most satisfying occurrence to emerge from our pandemic-induced discipline was that all of a sudden *everyone was washing their hands properly*. Hallelujah.

It was in 1847, on an obstetrics ward in Vienna, that a young Hungarian physician called Ignaz Semmelweis first observed the link between doctors performing autopsies on cadavers and the deaths of the mothers they also cared for on neighbouring maternity wards. He concluded that the simple act of hand-washing was an essential weapon in the fight against infection control, and if the doctors had only washed their hands when transitioning between wards then bacteria would not have passed from cadaver to mother, and many deaths might have been avoided. Up until the arrival of Covid-19 into our society, we as a human race had had a generous 173 years to digest and put into regular practice this basic scientific fact, and yet somehow it appeared that every other person on the planet had forgotten to think about and act upon this laughably simple health-preserving certainty multiple times each day, and therefore had to be reminded of its necessity by way of daily bulletins on our national news. A year or two before the pandemic, I stood in one of the longest queues for a toilet I have ever seen during the interval of an even longer play, and watched with utter incredulity as almost half of the people using the two tiny cubicles didn't bother to wash their hands on exiting. I tried to keep a mental note of each place that these offenders touched on the bathroom door, so as to avoid touching it myself on my own spotlessly clean departure, but it became too much to remember as I pictured them filtering back out into the theatre and touching handrails, backs of seats, regular doors, bar-tops. Not to mention the locks, flushes and seats in the cubicles themselves. Surely this constant stream of medically endorsed and very public supplication to wash our hands would finally and permanently rid society of not only Covid, but also help to eliminate other seasonal illnesses for good, too? Not as simple as that, I realise, but for months afterwards the instances of many contagious infections, for example flu and – most significantly for me – norovirus, did in in fact reduce dramatically, and in turn, so did my anxiety.

At this point it might be worth mentioning that acting as a profession is not the ideal bedfellow to OCD. It is a life fraught with uncertainty. At times completely wonderful, but in equal measure it involves a large helping of displacement, loneliness, insecurity, failure and waiting. Oh, the waiting. A lifetime of waiting for the next job, unsure where you will be in a month or two from now, unsure how to budget or make yourself feel vaguely useful in the meantime. Covid provided a rare equilibrium in which many people, no matter the job, status or state of mind, couldn't work as they normally did – some unable to do anything at all – and so the sense that I *should* be doing more was replaced by a knowledge that I *couldn't* be doing more, and so, for the first time in a long while, I was actually quite relaxed.

I felt as if I had been banging on the window of a house for twenty years, looking in from outside, desperately trying to alert an oblivious soul within to their impending doom. It seemed as though, finally, the rest of the world understood the implications of contagious illnesses, and could perhaps even begin to imagine what it was like to live with their own nest of scorpions. At last, they had turned to see me, by now exhausted and not entirely able to remember why I was banging in the first place, but overwhelmed with relief that my efforts had not been in vain.

However, this time, the scorpions had burrowed deep. I searched and searched but there was no sign of my nest. I slept deeply and dreamlessly, and thought often of this Zen proverb:

Before enlightenment, chop wood, carry water,
After enlightenment, chop wood, carry water.

In this moment of global existential crisis, I found the best thing I could do for some peace of mind was to try and take care of the small things. The everyday errands that sustain us and give us purpose ... Whilst I focused on the small things and let the grand worries dissolve into the background, my very own small things appeared to have left me, noiselessly and without warning. I relished the solitude and even began to dread the inevitable end to this blur of repetitive nothingness. Casting my mind back to that period of childhood chronic fatigue, I remembered how hopeless I found those endless days of monotony, navigating my peculiar months of exhausted repetition, and the irony was not lost of me. How familiarity feels good to us, even when it is not good *for* us ...

Psychasthenia is a term that is no longer used diagnostically in psychiatry but was once classified as a condition not too dissimilar to obsessive compulsive disorder. Nowadays it is a defunct term regarded as a mental condition that was conceived of before the onset of experimental psychology. Phobias, obsessions and compulsions were all symptoms attributed to patients. Concentration, self-criticism, fatigue and indecision were also factors, and at one stage Carl Jung used the 'psychasthenic' personality model as a prototype for his definition of introversion. German–Swiss psychiatrist Karl Jaspers described it as a 'diminution of psychic energy', which promotes daydreaming and withdrawal from the world – exacerbating the situation tenfold, of course.

There was an essay written by French scholar Roger Caillois in the mid-1930s that focused upon the relationship between psychasthenia and mimicry in nature. He theorised that mimicry in the animal world (a praying mantis transforming to resemble a leaf or a twig, for example) could not convincingly be attributed to a defensive strategy alone. As many predators hunt only by smell and frequently under the cover of nightfall – rendering the aesthetic disguise theory useless in the aforementioned scenarios – he determined that there was another reason for this impulse to camouflage. It was governed, he said, by 'a veritable *lure of space*' rather than a desire to hide, and he believed a similar motivation to assimilate to one's environment or spatial surroundings could be seen in humans. In other words, there are certain instances when the pull to become, or blend in to, one's space can become too powerful to resist, and whether it was intended or not, one loses the ability to feel or be seen.

Caillois goes on to state that psychasthenia is a form of this 'depersonalisation through assimilation into space' and can lead to a loss of one's sense of reality as well as one's sense of self. Fading into the background as a way of renouncing life. And there is no more perfect environment to induce this sense of psychasthenia than the conditions created by the Covid-19 lockdowns. In no time at all I found myself sympathising with and even enjoying these transformations practised by the likes of tiger moths and scarlet kingsnakes. I became a ghost floating through my own life, observing but no longer taking part. I felt a sense of achievement at the temporary loss of my compulsions, but also a sense of loss over the parts of myself that had gone missing, the more complex elements that made up what I knew to be 'me'.

The months of fear, death and uncertainty that the Covid-19 pandemic thrusted upon us gave me an unprecedented glimpse into the mind of someone living without OCD. A freedom. A clarity of mind. I could turn off a tap without going back to check it. I could go for a walk without photographing the contents of my apartment first. I could even get a decent night's sleep for once. Now that a highly contagious disease was spreading rapidly around the world, feasting on anyone and everyone no matter their walk of life – what else was there to actually legitimately worry about? The worst possible thing that could happen *was* happening, and in order to cope with it, my mind and body – along with many other people's minds and bodies – went into total shutdown. Perhaps I too readily allowed myself to disengage. Foolishly believing that because the scorpions disappeared for a short window of time, the answer was to starve myself of social contact, to flush them out and to avoid any future situation that might cause them to return. It was too easy to become a purposeless blob of indifference, to succumb to the temptation to lock myself away and bask in this blissful lack of responsibility.

But, as the virus diminished and the vaccine gave us back some semblance of power, society started to open up again and life continued to move forward, carefully and oh-so-slowly. I had to readjust to this new normal alongside everyone else around me, and once again began to hear the *tap-tap* of tiny feet returning diligently back to their nest, like birds returning from a summer migration. The idea of correspondence in any form disturbed my sleep. I would lie awake and look at the growing backlog of unanswered messages, check my alarm clock sixteen times to counteract the fear. My mind played tricks on me, convincing me that the hob was on, the tap was still running, the online supermarket delivery driver had been sick in his car and had touched my shopping bags with his infected hands … It was much safer inside, where I knew my parameters. Just me and the cat and the scorpions.

The local cemetery, pre- and post-pandemic, has always been one of my favourite places to walk and think and talk. A good friend sent me a message some weeks into the cautious reopening of society, as bubbles expanded and possibilities started to emerge, asking if I wanted to stroll amongst the graves whilst we caught up after so long without seeing one another. He knew the lure of this offer and in spite of my burgeoning anxiety at stepping back out into the world, I accepted the invitation, knowing, even so, that I would have to be ready thirty or maybe forty minutes earlier to allow for my apartment-departure routine. I felt a sense of responsibility to all those people that we'd lost to this devastating virus, to grab opportunities with both hands, no matter how much it filled me with dread. My scorpions clustered, laying the groundwork for a new start, a new routine, as I held in my mind a quote from Caillois's essay 'Mimicry and Legendary Psychasthenia'. A warning I try my best not to forget:

'Beware: whoever pretends to be a ghost will eventually turn into one.'

And so I stood up from my seat to begin my routine, phone poised in camera mode ready to catalogue my full breadth of physical evidence, and set off for the graveyard to walk amongst the dead, feeling very much alive.

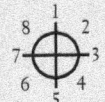

FRONT DOOR RITUAL

☒ Close and lock the front door.

☒ Pull at the door's handle for a count of 8, to make sure it is firmly closed.

$$1, 2, 3, 4, 5, 6, 7, 8.$$

☒ Push against the door for a count of 8, to make sure it can't be pushed open.

$$1, 2, 3, 4, 5, 6, 7, 8.$$

☒ Pull the door for a count of 8.

$$1, 2, 3, 4, 5, 6, 7, 8.$$

☒ Push the door for a count of 8.

$$1, 2, 3, 4, 5, 6, 7, 8.$$

☒ Pull the door for a count of 8.

$$1, 2, 3, 4, 5, 6, 7, 8.$$

☒ Push the door for a count of 8.

$$1, 2, 3, 4, 5, 6, 7, 8.$$

☒ Pull the door for a count of 8.

$$1, 2, 3, 4, 5, 6, 7, 8.$$

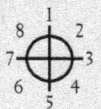

☒   Push the door for a count of 8.

          1, 2, 3, 4, 5, 6, 7, 8.

☒   Continue until you are satisfied it is closed.

☒   Ritual must be completed very rapidly and quietly, to avoid arousing suspicion that you are either:

> *breaking into a house that isn't yours; or*
> *losing your marbles.*

Chapter Eight

NUCLEAR

'Scorpions occur in a vast array of different environments
that put it in proximity to the most severe extremes of
atmospheric radiation on Earth.'

Tommy Rodriguez, 'A Possible Glimpse at the Role of
Naturally-Ocurring Radiation as a Contributing Factor to
Genetic Variance among Populations of Living Organisms'

In a year nestled somewhere amidst the late 2010s, I find myself back in my therapist's office for our first session in several months. This time, unlike every other time, I am sitting with my back to the clock, which ticks softly behind my head as I wait for the sound of the door opening and closing upstairs, followed by the leisurely patter of feet descending towards the calmest room on Earth. But she takes me by surprise and glides in noiselessly, giving herself a generous moment to assess the situation. The door must be oiled regularly, I think, to ensure seamless, unstartling transitions between rooms.

'Why are you sitting there?' she asks, a Mona Lisa smile on her lips.

I laugh nervously, knowing I've been caught out.

'Oh, yeah,' I say too quickly, as if I'd forgotten. 'I realised over the last few months that I've been sitting in your seat this whole time!' I chuckle. She is careful not to join in.

'What makes you think that was my seat?' she challenges.

'Well, isn't it? You sit there so you can keep an eye on the clock above the client's head, and I'm supposed to sit here so I can look at the inspirational quotes on the wall behind you. I never noticed them before …'

Another unreadable smile crosses her lips. 'Go back to your original seat. Feels weird.'

I bound back over to my usual spot, certain that she is analysing both my choice to hijack her chair during every session I have attended up until this point *and* my decision to spontaneously renounce said chair in favour of the allocated client seat. By the time I've arranged myself back on the armchair in a self-consciously 'relaxed' position, I'm convinced she thinks I've got a superiority complex. She, on the other hand, is a picture of genuine relaxation; her feet tucked up beneath leopardprint legs, her long blonde hair loose over her shoulders, a tangle of gold chains wrapping her wrists and neck. She takes a sip of water and adjusts the box of tissues placed on the table next to her, clearly meant for whichever client is correctly sitting in the assigned chair that she is now adorning. (I never know what to call the people who come through these doors to seek help, myself included. 'Client' feels too formal. 'Patient' feels too passive and clinical. Therapee? 'Hello, I'm the therapee, here for my therapy.' Too confusing, perhaps.) Her large blue eyes look directly through me to the writhing swarm of scorpions beneath. They look back at her, for a rare moment completely still.

'How have you been?' she begins.

At first, I didn't really want to see a therapist. It felt self-indulgent, like I didn't have the right to make someone sit through my particular litany of issues. There can be a misconception, which I bought in to as a teenager, that doing therapy means you have failed at the fundamental act of existing. I was in my mid-twenties when I finally swallowed my pride and began searching for a therapist. I was adamant that I wanted to see an old man. I didn't want a young man, in case I immediately fell in love with him. I didn't want an older woman, who might try to mother me. And I definitely didn't want a young woman, who might as well (in my mind) occupy the same position as one of my close friends. No, I wanted my therapist to be the caricature of an old Victorian gentleman: wise, unemotional and posing no threat to what I perceived as my susceptible psychological state. An Albert Einstein type who could give me a simple scientific solution to 'nip it all in the bud' and send me on my way. The search didn't quite go to plan, however, and led me straight into the arms of a woman no more than eight years my senior, who was everything I thought I didn't want and could not have been a better fit for me. What the hell did I know.

After around eighteen months of therapy, I took a break – under the pretence that my brain had been restored to its factory settings – only to return some months later with a different goal. This time my focus was more specific. I had sent her what I thought was a pretty well-constructed email.

To: Thezza
Subject: Availability?

Hi *****
Hope you're well?
Was wondering if you had any availability to see
me in the next couple of weeks and do a spot of
hypnotherapy for the old OCD?

Tuppence

She was in my contact list as 'Thezza' for the same
reason that I found it near impossible to say 'my therapist' aloud to anyone without doing so in a sickeningly
nasal Californian accent. I didn't take myself seriously. I'd
written several drafts of the email, in which 'a spot of' and
'the old' had not featured, before deciding upon the final
edit. I'd put them in to give myself a casual air. To let it
be known that I was in control of the situation and would
only require a mere nudge in the direction of sanity. The
rest could be solved with a smattering of hypnotherapy,
something I had fantasised about as being a cure-all
for basically all psychological afflictions without really
knowing anything about it beyond what I had learned
from the movies. I would sit, or ideally lie, on a comfortable sofa whilst Thezza murmured calming words at me
from across the room until I fell into a half-sleep within
which I would be processing healing images and subcon-

sciously learning strategies that would help me not to be terrified of throwing up the next time I was conscious. As it happens, we never actually tried hypnotherapy, so that fantasy has remained firmly intact. Once I found my way back into her chair, it somehow didn't seem so important. All I really wanted to do was *talk*.

My scorpions have been pretty tenacious over the years, akin to those found in the wild, which are one of only a few species that have survived exposure to nuclear radiation. Extinguishing them is a multi-faceted mission. There are few natural things that can seriously damage a scorpion. Their capacity for self-protection being so great, an urban myth was born to fully encapsulate the indestructible nature of this robust little creature. It is said that if you place a scorpion in a circle of fire so high that it cannot escape, it will take its own life by repeatedly stinging itself rather than die a gruesome natural death. This is not actually true. As is the case with most arthropods, a scorpion is unable to regulate its own body temperature, and so as the fire causes its body to grow hotter and hotter, the scorpion becomes dehydrated, the pain and suffocation throwing its stinger into spasm – creating the illusion that it is stinging itself to death, when really it simply overheats and eventually dries out, the life evaporating slowly and painfully from its tiny form. For me to attempt to destroy my own scorpions has sometimes felt as if it carries this same inevitable risk of self-destruction. They just keep coming back to life.

My first attempt to kill them was the NHS-prescribed cognitive behavioural therapy sessions I attended the year after leaving drama school. Cognitive behavioural therapy (CBT) is a form of talking therapy in which you are given ways to help reduce negative thought patterns. Rather than exploring your past for answers as to why your mind might be behaving in a particular way, it simply deals with your current problems and offers practical solutions for managing them on a daily basis. It has been proven to be one of the most successful ways to treat OCD, but for me personally it felt hopeless to fight a disorder that was resistant to logic *with* logic. It could have been that I didn't give the treatment enough time to work its magic, but looking back I think perhaps I wasn't ready to begin that kind of treatment. The type of treatment that gave you homework in the form of logging your own menacing thoughts each week with the intention of replacing those thoughts with more positive ones, and which also filled me with the constant fear that I was going to be made to watch people throw up in order to graduate from my programme. I was so terrified of being made to face my fears that I filled out all of the worksheets given to me by my practitioner in a way that gave the impression that I was able to cure myself of intrusive thought cycles. I ticked all the right boxes and agreed dutifully when asked if the sessions were helping, giving the performance of my life as a young woman who was overcoming her compulsive behaviour and disordered way of thinking. I couldn't bear to disappoint my enthusiastic young therapist, to look into her enormous brown eyes and tell her the simple truth. That I was scared of what it might require of me to make myself better, and that I didn't feel that this kind of logic-driven, behaviour-focused approach was the right fit for me. And so, after a block of eight arduous sessions, I was discharged from her care and my GP was informed that the treatment had been successful. Case closed. Or so they thought.

The next assassination attempt on the scorpions came around three years later, when my anxiety increased substantially and the physical effects of that began to take their toll on my body. I was living alone at the time and finding it impossible to get any sleep due to the panic attacks I was experiencing on a semi-regular basis. I would often wake myself in the early hours of the morning, sweaty and unable to breathe properly, a sharp pain across my chest. The traumatic and perplexing thing about panic attacks is that when you are inside of one, they feel completely unconnected to an emotionally or psycho-logically driven thought process. The feeling is entirely physical. If you have never had one before, it can feel like you are dying. I was so worried that the cumulative effect of these panic attacks would put such stress on my body that I would have an actual heart attack, and scared myself into seeking a more chemical solution to help control what was happening to my body. Despite my intense fear of sickness or developing any disease that could potentially kill me,

I have always been one of those frustrating people who waits until the headache is almost blinding them before they take a painkiller. This doesn't stem from a mistrust of the medication itself, but that I want to feel the exact strength and nature of the pain as it is occurring, so that I can assess the seriousness of the situation at all times and remain in control of my own perception of the pain. So, I waited until the physical toll of anxiety – the rapid heartbeat, the breathlessness, the chest pain, the stomach cramps, the insomnia – became unbearable, and I decided to return to the first solution that had been offered to me as a teenager.

When treating obsessive compulsive disorder, the medication that has been proven to treat symptoms successfully above all others are serotonin re-uptake inhibitors, or SRIs. The same type of medication that is prescribed to treat depression. Serotonin is a chemical used by the brain as a messenger, so if you are not producing enough serotonin, then the nerves in your brain might not be communicating effectively with the rest of your body and your brain cannot function as it should. Interestingly, serotonin deficiency is also a significant clinical finding in patients with chronic fatigue syndrome, the illness I developed as a child. There is still a lack of understanding as to exactly *why* these drugs help to improve OCD symptoms, but after decades of research, they have shown themselves to be the most effective. At first, I was given a strong anti-anxiety medication called diazepam.

I didn't know much about it, but was alerted to its potency immediately when I was prescribed only four small tablets 'for emergencies'. I wasn't quite sure what constituted an emergency, but when I began to have a panic attack before boarding a long-haul plane journey, I seized the moment and took the first of my four little life jackets. It kicked in remarkably quickly and I spent the duration of the flight in a drowsy, soupy euphoria that allowed me to use the plane toilet without having a meltdown, to ignore the individual back-stories of all the other passengers onboard, and to finally get some much-needed slumber. So what if the edges were blurred?

It didn't take long for my definition of 'emergency' to become worryingly loose, and I realised why I had been given so few tablets. They are undeniably moreish. Or at least the effect of them is. There was no opportunity for me to develop an addiction to the medication, having been given very little of it, but I understood immediately how dangerous the effectiveness of drugs like these can be if used in the wrong way. Addiction was just as frightening to me as disease, and so going forward I was prescribed an antidepressant called fluoxetine, commonly known as Prozac. The doctor prescribing it warned me that it could make me feel worse before I started to feel better, as it takes a while for the body to process the new chemical levels in the blood. His warning turned out to be well needed. I spent the best part of two weeks over the Christmas holidays that year with increased anxiety, shakiness, heart palpitations and sleeplessness, and then, all of a sudden, without my even noticing, the worst had passed and the drugs began to take effect. When the new year arrived, I felt calmer, more in control, less enslaved to the scorpions. I could sleep through the night and my panic attacks stopped completely. I felt stabilised for the first time in a long time.

Although my physical symptoms had improved, I was still aware of a hum of activity continuing inside my head. Just because I couldn't see or feel the effects of the scorpions, it didn't mean they weren't still there, chipping away at my neural pathways, weaving new and complex thoughts into the bedrock of my brain. After a blissful two years of feeling something close to normal on the outside, I decided to take advantage of this momentum and put everything into attacking my little monsters from the inside too. Whilst the medication helped my body to feel calm and strong, I began my first foray into psychotherapy, or talking therapy.

Whilst I sat in the chair clearly meant for my therapist, I revisited the idea that there is probably not a person on Earth who wouldn't benefit from trying therapy. Good therapy, in my experience, should feel akin to good acting. Totally invisible. If you can see the thoughts or the seams of the performance, then you lose faith in its reality. The same goes for the delicate dance that is the relationship between therapist and therapee.© Both require an exchange of trust, openness and discovery. Someone who is guarding their scorpions close can smell the faintest whiff of dishonesty, and so the therapist often has to earn their trust. Although I was already treating the physical side of OCD, I wanted to address my disordered thoughts and where they came from. My therapist didn't make notes during our sessions, she just listened and shared and suggested. She calculated when to hug me and when not to hug me, she learned my tells and my insecurities, my happy places and my points of conflict. I realised over time that I had for most of my life underestimated the power of talking. As this slow and steady process began to blunt the pincers and neutralise the stings, my therapist suggested making steps towards coming off my medication. It had been just over two years that I'd been taking the tablets; they were so much a part of my daily routine that I had almost forgotten why I was taking them. They sat alongside my contraceptive pill and my fair-weather omega-3s as one more ingredient in a pre-breakfast cocktail. I no longer felt any change when I took them, just normality, so I was feeling daunted by the idea of saying goodbye to my crutch and fending for myself again. Would the panic attacks come back? Would talking about my scorpions really be enough to keep them at bay?

The idea was to support my coming off the tablets with talking therapy, replacing my need to take them with therapy alone. When I had first returned to my therapist I had been taking them for two years, but within six months of restarting our sessions I had stopped. Coming off was, for me, nothing compared to starting the tablets, which I attribute in part to continuing therapy at my own pace whilst slowly lowering my dosage until there was nothing left to consume. The scorpions were still there, but those years breathed space into my crowded mind. It was no longer a cramped and festering mass, but an open passageway for the scorpions to pass through. Sometimes there are more than others, sometimes they get lost in that excess of space and I don't feel them for weeks on end, and sometimes there is a blockage – a lone scorpion stuck in the outer reaches of my mind, leading all the others to the same place until the pressure builds and I must find my own ways to set them free.

In Hindu tradition scorpion bites are known to have been treated by the recitation of mantras. There is a special mantra which consists of counting from 100 back to 1, then repeating the whole count 108 times. Allegedly, this mantra is said to work solely on Holi or Diwali festival days, or during solar or lunar eclipses. Only an obsessive can appreciate how satisfying this kind of specificity can be ...

My rituals and routines function in much the same way as these mantras. Through counting or checking or touching, I soothe the anxious energy in my body and calm the negative thoughts until that thrumming swarm is reduced to a distant scuttle. When the rituals don't satisfy my obsessions, then I take photographs to assure myself.

When I can't assure myself, I look to others to reassure me. When I can't be reassured, I wash my hands, I avoid people, I don't leave the house, I invent a new routine, a new bargain, a new unpleasant thought. And when the nest overwhelms me again, I return to my role as therapee.

Treatment is an ever-evolving process, as different for each person as it has been for me at every stage of my life with OCD. Each avenue has provided me with something that I can choose to take with me, a new way of approaching those days when everything feels stuck. A sense of relief that there is help out there, however the scorpions choose to surprise me. It is just a matter of asking for it.

To do:
Laundry
Shopping (red wine)
* *A spot of the old hypnotherapy*

Ode to Coleridge

Scorpions, scorpions everywhere,
And no will left to think;
Scorpions, scorpions everywhere,
Their prehistoric stink.

How very deep they dig: O God!
Why won't they let me be!
These slimy things with hellish stings
Have taken part of me.

About, about, by day they roam,
Then horror comes at night;
Their pincers like a devil's horn,
Their poison burning bright.

And in my dreams, I can't be sure
If they have plagued me so.
But when I wake, they've followed me
To the land of flesh and bone.

Chapter Nine

WARDING

'By the side of the scorpion do not come,
by the side of the snake spread your bed and sleep.'

Arabic proverb

Sometimes I like to time-travel by waving to myself in the future and then remembering to wave back when I have reached my intended destination. I have already finished writing this book, but you are still in the act of reading it. It has nine chapters, a prologue and an epilogue. Which is, of course, an *odd* number of chapters.

Without realising, I had been resisting losing or adding certain chapters because it would disrupt my desire to create a book with an *even* number of chapters. So unnerving was the idea of writing a book in nine chapters that I have taken it upon myself to add another as a preventative measure against the wrath of the scorpions. Chapter Nine became Chapter Ten, and this has become Chapter Nine.

So here it is, over before it has begun.

An utterly pointless little wave to my unsettled future self.

And a gruntled one back.

Chapter Ten

(RE)BIRTH

*'Consider the scorpion as it sinks into apolysis, when
the epidermal cells gradually separate from the hard old
exoskeleton. A new cuticle begins to form, and the creature
within agitates, thrusting back and forth until the old
integumentary shell cracks. It squeezes out, reborn.'*

Justin E.H. Smith, 'The Art of Molting'

A rogue blob of tomato sauce has fallen from my pizza onto the bed. I should probably clean it up but I don't really have the energy after the marathon I have just endured, and there's so much blood saturating the sheets I'm not sure there is any point. I have just given birth to my daughter and I am ravenous, barely stopping for breath between slices as I feel the loop and tug of stitches being woven into my flesh, see the duck and bob of a midwife's head appearing between my legs, deep in concentration. In my free arm I cradle an impossibly tiny, impossibly intricate human form who has taken the best part of a day to enter into this world, arriving in a heatwave so intense I had to stop four times on the short walk from the car park to the hospital entrance. I keep looking at her, disbelieving. She is more perfect than perfect. I am swimming in endorphins and bursting with love for everyone and everything around me: my partner with a grin the size of Antarctica, the woman who has been diligently sewing my perineum for the last forty-five minutes, the terrible slice of pizza I am inhaling. I think about all the things that had scared me about having a child previously. *What if I get severe morning sickness and I vomit every day for nine months? There will be no escape until it's over. What will happen when my child gets sick? Will I be able to cope or care for her? Can I raise a child without ever visiting a soft play and entrenching myself in other people's germs?* Here in the birth centre, flushed with love and exhaustion, I cannot imagine ever feeling anxious again. Each breath of my recovery makes me feel stronger. Invincible. I begin to contemplate the idea of a rebirth. I *wish* for a shedding of old uncomfortable skin, to free my scorpions and leave them here in a little box, to keep the newborns company before they are released out into the world. This time, I think, I might really be able to do it.

Several weeks later, we are going for a walk on a hot afternoon in late summer. Around half a mile from our house my partner turns to me and says, 'Hey, you know you didn't check the door when you left?'

'What?' I answer, my brain not quite catching up.

'The door, you didn't check the door after you locked it. You didn't do your routine. I noticed it as soon as we left the house, but I didn't want to say anything.' He smiles.

I start to retrace my steps and realise he's right. I have no memory of leaving the house whatsoever, I was so focused on our daughter. He can see the cogs begin to turn as I try my hardest to remember if I actually did lock the door, or even close it, then grabs both of my arms tightly and says, 'No, don't think about it! This is great!'

I don't even have any photographs to check. We aren't *so* far away from home, I calculate. My usually snail-like walking pace is subconsciously kicked up a notch, and I shuffle home as fast as my healing body will allow. Can I really have killed my demons?

It would be wonderful if that were the end of it. Not only the end of the book, but of my whole journey with OCD, gone as quickly as it arrived – never to be seen again. Confirmation to the contrary came in the dairy aisle at big Sainsbury's after just over eight months of being a parent. After managing to both keep her alive and survive the perils of baby vomit unscathed, I felt pretty proud of myself. The vomit of months gone by had remained firmly on the GOOD VOMIT list by adhering to the standard rules of milky infant regurgitation, but this time was different. I was on my way over to the cheeses, our daughter strapped to my body, when I heard a strange sound bubbling below my chin. I looked down and found that she was staring at me, a confused expression on her face. We locked eyes and she smiled, as if surprised that I also happened to be here in aisle 23, buying cheese at the same exact moment as her. I smiled back and she laughed in the adorable way babies do, then made a short, sharp sound like a computer game avatar powering up for a blow, and projectile vomited all over my chest. It was a flawless shot, carried out at extreme close range, and as each millisecond passed I could feel the liquid running down my body, into my bra, down the back of my neck, collecting inside my belly button. Immediately I blew all the air out of my mouth and began to jog frantically between the aisles looking for my partner, who I found a few minutes later by the noodles. All the while our daughter giggled hysterically, like my increased speed signalled some kind of game that she seemed to enjoy but didn't really understand. Prior to this, her being sick had always been chalked up to her developing stomach being too full of milk or following through on an enthusiastic burp. I knew immediately that this was illness-related: the sheer amount that came out of her mouth, the force at which it ejected itself from her little body, the smell of it.

'Quick! Help! She's just thrown up on me!'

'OK. Well, that's OK. Here, pass her to me while you clean yourself up.' He reaches out his hands and takes her from the carrier. I marvel silently at the lack of flinch or grimace when a little pool of vomit that has been trapped between her and my body drips down onto his fingers.

'I think she must have a bug – she's never sick like this!' I declare.

He looks doubtful. 'No, she doesn't, but it's only because she just ate and she was strapped to you. Her stomach was probably pressing up against yours as you were walking and it made her sick.'

It's not a bad hypothesis, but doubting this kind of baseless claim has always kept me safe in the past, so I'm not taking any chances. I sprint to the supermarket toilet with my hands held awkwardly above my waist about a foot away from my body, fingers spread like they're coated in Novichok. About fifteen minutes later, after repeatedly washing my hands and chest, and soaking my dress to remove most of the vomit, I return to the checkout to find our daughter happily gurgling away in the seat of the trolley.

'See! She's fine. Happy as Larry,' says my partner, dialling up the positivity to convince me of his confidence in the matter. Larry. Unfortunate reference, I think, unable to shake Dr Makison Booth's simulated vomiting machine, Vomiting Larry, from my mind. We quickly pay and steer the trolley to our car, but all the while I'm studying her for signs that it's more than just a touch of indigestion. She's loaded into the car, along with the shopping, for the short drive home. I take the wheel so I can keep an eye on her in the rear-view mirror, whilst my partner tries his best to distract me with conversation. Two minutes in, just as I am beginning to relax, I spot her eyes glaze over and suddenly she looks very tired. We haven't been driving long enough for the engine to lull her to sleep and she isn't due a nap for another few hours. I know exactly what's happening.

'She's going to be sick again. She looks … strange,' I announce, fighting to keep my eyes on the road.

'She doesn't look strange! She looks tired,' he says, without looking. Her head flops forward and she spits out her dummy, and at this point I notice that all the colour has drained from her cheeks.

'I don't have a mask with me!' I blurt out. I have got into the habit of hiding face masks about the house and in several of my bags in case I'm at any given time surprised by a vomiting incident – the only souvenir from the days of Covid-19 that I've been compelled to keep. There are none in the car, and so I bow down to the scorpions to stop her vomiting, at least until we get home and are within leaping distance of an FFP2. And then it happens, as I knew it would. An almighty retch from the back seat and Happy Larry vomits forcefully onto the chair in front of her. Twice.

I panic and, without thinking, pull haphazardly over to the kerb, the car partially blocking the road with its aggressive angle, and eject myself, leaving the door wide open with the engine still running. I know I look like a madwoman, but I don't care. Thankfully there is no traffic in this part of town. The passenger door swings open and out jumps my partner.

'OhGodshe'sbeensickshemusthaveavirusthere'snowaywewon'tcatchitwhatdowedo?!' My words come out in one long stream of consciousness.

'Just stay calm. I'll get her.' I hear a double splash of vomit hitting the gravel and I try my hardest not to breathe. 'Whoa, that's a lot of puke,' my partner observes. He takes her in his arms and begins walking. I can see strings of vomit dribbling from her mouth as she bounces along on his hip. 'I'll walk the rest of the way home; you drive the car back.'

Home is only a two-minute walk away, and so off he sets as I hesitate at the thought of having to get back inside the car with two festering pools of vomit, filling the car with infectious particles ready to glide effortlessly into my throat. I close my eyes and see the elevator doors from *The Shining* open in slow motion and release not a river of blood, but a gushing torrent of vomit heading straight for my orifices. I need to act quickly. From outside the car, I put my hand on the edge of the driver's door to roll down all four windows simultaneously, so I don't have to breathe the concentrated air of contagion. I take a step away from the car and inhale deeply, breathing in as much fresh air as my lungs can take, then launch myself into the driver's seat, release the handbrake and drive full speed to the space outside our front door. They will arrive not long after me, so I have just enough time to locate the bleach, run a bath, prepare some plastic bags and find a face mask. I glance down the road to check their status as I refill my lungs with clean air, and I can see them walking towards me in the distance. Overwhelmed with shame at regarding my own daughter with the same fear as an approaching zombie, I scurry inside to set up my own personal hygiene laboratory. But in the back of my mind, after years of research and mental preparation, I realise the terrifying truth: I have probably already caught it. A direct hit to the chest, so close to my mouth and nose, certainly less than a two-metre distance ... I didn't stand a chance. Nevertheless, I set to work turning my home into a makeshift hospital.

It only took around twelve hours for the symptoms to appear. I had expected it to be longer. Despite my desperate overnight appeal to the scorpions, I began to get stomach pains the next day. A fever developed some hours later, along with some nausea, but I was never *actually* sick. Miserable as I was, I thanked the scorpions for allowing me this relief, for sparing me the horror of vomiting. Logically speaking, one can assume that the underdeveloped immune systems of children manifest a virus in a more extreme way than the version transmitted to the hardier adults around them. But here lies the problem with OCD: I can never be sure that if I hadn't 'appealed' to my scorpions, and promised them rituals and loyalty in return for their protection from illness, that I wouldn't have gotten sicker. Looking from the outside, one would hope the lesson learned was that, although I did catch the illness, it wasn't as bad for me as expected, and it was such a small insignificant moment within the wider context of my life that it just doesn't make sense to dedicate a remarkable amount of time obsessing about it. One would *hope*. The lesson I took from it, however, was this: I need a VOMIT BOX. Not a box to vomit into, but a box with which to defend myself against vomit. After further research and a considerable online shopping stint, I put together the following kit:

1 *giant plastic box (labelled* VOMIT)
6 *pairs of extra-strong rubber gloves*

2 boxes of 50pcs FFP2 surgical-grade face masks
6 bottles thick bleach
4 bottles bleach spray

The kit lives in my bathroom, hidden from sight but within instant reach for the emergency event of any future stomach bugs invading our home. Not quite the rebirth I was counting on. How can something as life-changingly momentous as birthing a child not demote my mental health to far below the average worry on my priority list? It is a tough pill to swallow, admitting the shame of letting a disorder hijack your ability to care for your own sick child.

The question that has often confronted me since the birth of my scorpions remains at the forefront of my mind: is it nature or nurture that coaxed them into existence? There is evidence to suggest that obsessive compulsive disorder does run in families, but there is also an environmental factor to consider. It can be said that whilst the genes 'load the gun', one's environment 'pulls the trigger'. Just because OCD may be present in your genetic make-up, that doesn't mean that it will ever manifest without an external stressor to ignite the onset of symptoms.

François de La Rochefoucauld, a seventeenth-century French writer and nobleman, expressed so perfectly in his seminal work *Maximes* the delicate balance of recovery and relapse when considering the complexities of the mind:

> The defects and faults of the mind are like wounds in the body; after all imaginable care has been taken to heal them up, still there will be a scar left behind, and they are in continual danger of breaking the skin and bursting out again.

Looking towards the future, I consider what I will tell our daughter about my little companions. Their presence in our home will be difficult to hide, as hard as I might try, and although they are creatures of the dark, she will be watching. Always watching, whether I see it or not. So, what of genetics? Will those same scorpions one day, when I am distracted or elsewhere, move to set up home in her own unspoiled mind?

Perhaps they are already there.

Epilogue

TOXINS

'These pharmacological properties of scorpion-derived bioactive molecules include antimicrobial, immunosuppressive, bradykinin-potentiating, analgesic, and anticancer effects among others ... there may indeed be great promise in exploiting the benefits of scorpion toxins.'

Shirin Ahmadi et al., 'Scorpion Venom: Detriments and Benefits'

Scorpions can be deadly, yet they have provided us with a great many remarkable things. They can glow in the dark, survive for up to a year without food, and they have given us the building blocks with which to create some life-altering medications.

From South Asia to North Africa the antidote most commonly used against scorpion poison is an oil 'pickled' with scorpions themselves, which is extracted by frying their bodies over extreme heat. Similarly, in 1950s Afghanistan there was a medical practitioner who specialised in curing skin diseases with ingredients made from scorpions and reptiles, but who ultimately died from a snake bite in the mid-1960s, such was the risk of fraternising with these creatures. So when the scorpions have nested and refuse to leave our side, is there a way in which we can we live with them or even *use* them to help us?

There are times when my arthropod friends all but disappear for a while, but I have never been able to shake them for good. They have shaped who I am for so many years that it is hard to separate them from my sense of self. My therapist once said that the things that are familiar to us often feel most comfortable, so we feel safe with them, reassured by what we know. But, she said, familiarity doesn't always mean that something is right or good; in fact it can often mean the opposite. I try to carry that notion with me, that knowledge of my scorpions. I can rely on them, I understand how they work, I know how to please them and they know how to influence me, but this safety in familiarity is something I have to watch carefully. Are they my captors? Or am I theirs?

OCD at its worse can be debilitating and can prevent sufferers from living a happy, functioning life. It can require twenty-four-hour care and cost people their independence, their livelihoods and their relationships. At this end of the scale, the condition needs specialist help and cannot merely be monitored or managed. But what about the remaining percentage of us with obsessive compulsive disorder? Those who live outwardly functioning lives but struggle to maintain control of their complex thoughts and behaviours. For me, it feels as though the condition is always adapting to survive. One year it may respond to a certain type of treatment, whilst the next that same treatment has little effect. It can manifest in a way that you could never have predicted, forcing you to change how you see the world. Or it can accompany you quietly, like a gentle hum always vibrating somewhere in the background of daily life. For those times when I can hear the hum, I try my best to find that glow in the dark. During the most stressful or difficult periods I have always attempted to look for the drive within the control, the empathy within the over-analysis, the focus within the repetition. Sometimes I find each of these lights at the end of their respective tunnels, and sometimes they are nowhere to be seen.

For instance, I can push the limits of my anxiety to breaking point by researching and obsessing about illness; but as a result of an excessive concern for the state of my health, I have on occasion detected evidence of a condition far earlier than I ordinarily would have, and as a result have been able to remedy it before any troublesome symptoms began to appear. Studies show that people with health-focused OCD generally become ill much less often than the average, due to their preoccupation with avoiding contagion and washing their hands more than the average person, as well as being more likely to book frequent doctor appointments. Some with other manifestations of the condition are so dedicated to the finer details that they will not leave a job imperfectly done, and others are so concerned that something terrible will happen and prepare themselves accordingly that they become the only person you want to have around you in a moment of crisis. Finding benefits to these distressing behaviours or obsessions, however small, can help me to accept and manage my thought processes a little better. To be kinder to myself and see the nuances of OCD for what they are. It is dangerous to suggest that OCD is just a series of behaviours that can be utilised in a positive way when needed, but when things feel overwhelming it can help to hold on to any constructive traits within the mass of tangled thought.

In Greek mythology, the hunter Orion gloated to the goddess Artemis that he could kill every animal on Earth. Unimpressed by his arrogance, Artemis sent a scorpion to kill the hunter. It succeeded, and as a warning to mortals about the dangers of pride, the almighty Zeus raised both Orion and the scorpion to the heavens where their constellations can be seen across the world. They were placed on opposite sides of the sky, so whilst Orion can be seen hunting each winter, he flees thereafter as Scorpius rises in the summer months – the two never meeting again. In this story the scorpion represents the hero, an embodiment of strength, courage and power. In depictions of the scorpion in ancient East Asian art it is an emblem of protection, a ward against evil. Yet across much of contemporary Muslim folklore the scorpion is considered to be an 'underworld creature', a symbol of evil that inhabits hell itself. In Indo-Pakistani culture the scorpion is used as a metaphor for carnal desire and lust, the scorpion's sting a manifestation of the erect penis. And in the Mesopotamian poem the *Epic of Gilgamesh* a scorpion man and a scorpion woman, who guard the twin peaks of Mount Mashu at the edge of the world, are at first regarded as fearsome creatures, but later reveal themselves to be benevolent beings, granting Gilgamesh passage to continue his journey and warning him of the dangers along the way. With the same ambiguity and openness, my scorpions serve to both protect me and push me towards danger. Stripped of them, I would feel off balance, somehow incomplete. Yet all I want is for someone to take them from me, to lighten the load. A mother scorpion will carry up to three dozen young on her back before their first molt. I'm beginning to know how she feels.

Was Tennessee Williams right when he said that to kill all his demons might kill his angels too? I am not sure yet if I agree, but the reality is that I would have to eradicate the scorpions for good to truly know. The professional help I have received along the way has shown me ways to cope by myself when needed. It has allowed me to feel more confident about taking back control of my thoughts and to celebrate the strange and complicated minds belonging to the obsessive-compulsives of this world. Mental health affects everyone in some way, and, in an age when anxiety is more widespread than it has ever been before, one of the most important things is that we have access to help, to stories and examples of the ways in which we can manifest our struggles and begin to heal.

When I was growing up, and my scorpions were too, all I wanted was to know that I wasn't the only one. I wanted to hear and learn about other people who thought or acted as I did. I needed a figure to show me that a life with OCD is not a hopeless one. It is surmountable, with the right guidance and medical help, and whether my scorpions are hibernating or voraciously present, I have learned to live alongside them.

In the quieter moments, when my mind is calm and my body at rest, I close my eyes and conjure Serket, the Egyptian queen wearing her scorpion crown for all to see. The figure I longed for as a child, the icon who bridles and embraces her demons. An icon I can share with my daughter, whoever she may become. This figure stands before me, proud and afraid, defiant and vulnerable, a beast tamed and placid upon her head, never forgetting the sting suspended above, a breath away from danger.

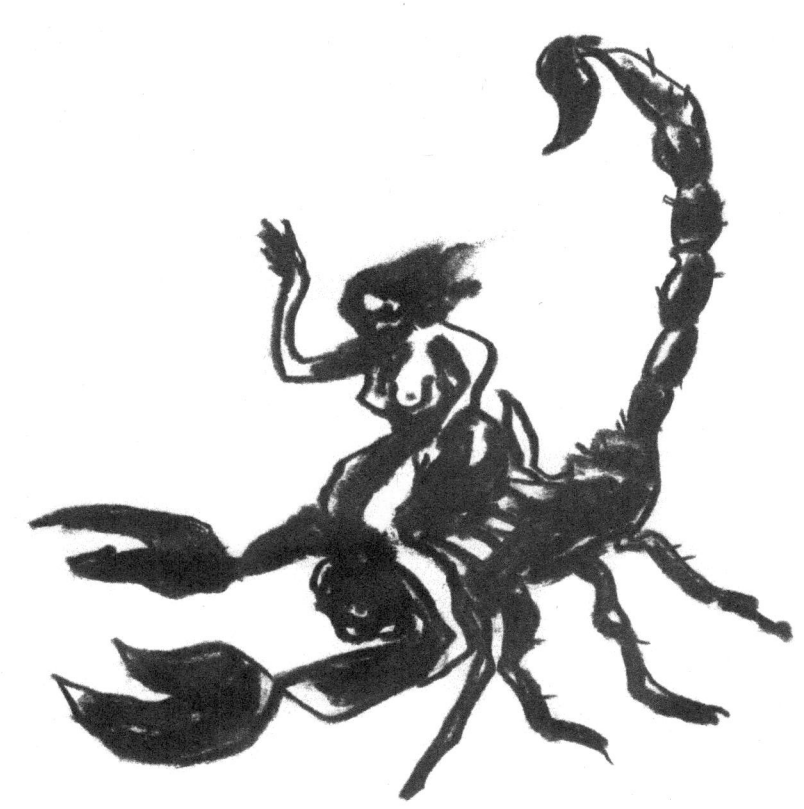

ACKNOWLEDGEMENTS

To Mum and Dad. Thank you doesn't really touch the sides...

For supporting me no matter which paths I took (even the questionable ones).

For believing I could do anything I put my mind to.

For your immeasurable love. I owe you everything.

To my family.

The Hobbit clan, thank you for making me see the funny side of everything.

My sister and brother (for being such massively important weirdos).

To my friends.

You know who you are. Few but fierce.

For always listening, understanding, turning up.

To Emmy, for showing me the way and for your special healing heart.

To Jane Finigan and everyone at Lutyens & Rubinstein.

Came for the agent, stayed for the friendship. Thank you for trusting me and spotting the seed I didn't know was there. Lucky me, being taken under that incomparable wing of yours. Thank you, Lisa Owens, for connecting the dots.

To my editor extraordinaire, Ru Merritt.

Cool as a cucumber. Smart as a button. Happy as Larry. Thank you for setting me free and guiding my words with the most delicate hand.

To all the brilliant minds of Ebury at Penguin Random House: editor Evangeline Stanford, publicist XXX, marketer XXX, text designer Jonathan Baker, copy editor Alice Brett, and proofreader XXX.

To Jesper Waldersten.

For making my book a thousand times cooler with your art. I am your number one fan.

To Måns. My eternal white rabbit.

The biggest heart and most exquisite mind in the universe.

Without you, none of this would be possible. You make me better, stronger, braver.

Jag älskar oss och den där fåniga lilla röda stolen.

You know the drill.

To my daughter. My beautiful girl. Nothing else matters.

Love books? Hate waste?
Then read on . . .

If you've finished with this proof but don't want to keep it, you unfortunately can't give it to charity or pass it on*. But, don't worry, you can recycle it.

Here's how:

Step One: if the cover, front or back, has any laminations, varnishes, or foils**, please tear it off and put it in your non-recycling rubbish.

Step Two: place the book in your recycling (after checking how your local recycling treats books at **recyclenow.com**).

You're done.

If you'd like to be greener still, then next time ask for a proof in a digital format.

We're making our books more recyclable

To find out more about our sustainability commitments including our journey to net zero, please visit greenpenguin.co.uk.

* They are not the final text and as such are available only for a limited time.

** These can contain metals and plastics.

SCORPIONS

A MEMOIR

Advance uncorrected proof copy
Not for resale or quotation
Rider • Published 27 February 2025 • £18.99
9781846048029 Hardback • 9781529923353 eBook
For publicity enquiries, please contact Jasleen Dhindsa on
JDhindsa@penguinrandomhouse.co.uk

SCORPIONS

TUPPENCE MIDDLETON

Rider, an imprint of Ebury Publishing
One Embassy Gardens, 8 Viaduct Gardens,
Nine Elms, London SW11 7BW

Rider is part of the Penguin Random House group of companies
whose addresses can be found at global.penguinrandomhouse.com

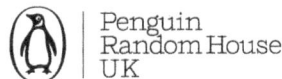

Penguin
Random House
UK

First published by Rider in 2025

www.penguin.co.uk

A CIP catalogue record for this book is available from the British Library

ISBN 9781846048029

Printed and bound in Great Britain by Clays Ltd, Elcograf S.p.A.

The authorised representative in the EEA is Penguin Random House Ireland,
Morrison Chambers, 32 Nassau Street, Dublin D02 YH68.

Penguin Random House is committed to a sustainable future for
our business, our readers and our planet. This book is made
from Forest Stewardship Council® certified paper.

For Toilethead